What people a

"I've known of and respected Dr. Z⌐ ⌐ ⌐ years. He is a true healer and teacher, and his comprehensive, holistic style of healthcare is ahead of its time."
—**Dr. Howard Cohn, DC**

"Anyone interested in finding or regaining health must read this book. *Misdiagnosed: The Adrenal Fatigue Link* is an inspiration!"
—**Dr. Aubry Tager, DC, CAFNI, BCIM**

"Get inspired to make good choices and live more healthfully, vibrantly, and youthfully with the tips and advice that Dr. Steven Zodkoy offers in his new book, *Misdiagnosed: The Adrenal Fatigue Link.*"
—**Sammy Pyon, DC**

"Dr. Steven Zodkoy shares from his heart and from his experience in this book. I believe *Misdiagnosed: The Adrenal Fatigue Link* bridges the gap in existing treatment methodologies for the veterans we serve."
—**Jack Downing, President/CEO, Soldier On**

"This book is for anyone serious about embracing a natural approach to an improved life—at any age."
—**Janet Bray Attwood, New York Times Bestseller & Co-author of *The Passion Test***

"With adrenal gland fatigue becoming more and more prevalent in today's society, I am so glad Dr. Zodkoy took the time to write this book, and you will be too!"
—**Dr. Steven Clarke, former chiropractic association president**

"As a mother of eight and a U.S. Marine, I have seen much across the physical and emotional spectrum. Of all that I have accomplished, one of the most significant would be to get you to trust what Dr. Zodkoy tells you. This is not a theory. I have experienced and seen the life-changing results time and again. Don't wonder if it works; it does. It is transformational. Don't wait."
—**Brigadier General Marcela Monahan, USMC**

Misdiagnosed

The Adrenal Fatigue Link

Misdiagnosed
The Adrenal Fatigue Link

By Dr. Steven Zodkoy

Book Cover design by Cathi Stevenson
www.BookCoverExpress.com

Interior Design by Rudy Milanovich
rudy@wizardvision.com

Book Edited by Maura Leon and Patrick Ennis

Front cover image © Nastco/iStockPhoto.com

ISBN: 978-0-9884471-1-0

Babypie Publishing
Waitsfield, VT
www.BabypiePublishing.com

Contents

Acknowledgements

I would like to express my gratitude to those who have helped me with this book and with my career:

To Melisa R., "Queen of the Little People," for finding the big editing errors

To my patients for believing in me and allowing me to guide them in their healing journey

To my office manager, Marie, for her support and excellent work

To my niece, Shaina, for helping with the research and patient interviews

To my publishers, Maura and Keith Leon, and their team for all that they did to help me get this book completed and into your hands...I trusted the process!

And finally, to Judy, Zoe, and Max...simply, I LOVE YOU... but, one of you a little more...you know who you are

Introduction

Are you tired of not feeling right? Would you like to feel more relaxed, calmer, and happier while living with less pain? Have you had enough of knowing there is something wrong with your body but not getting the answers you need from your physician? Are you starting to realize that something else needs to be done?

If you answered yes to any of these questions, then you are reading the right book!

I wrote this book for you, the reader, and not for your physician. I have taken some minor liberties with the technical wording and purposely kept the medical jargon and clinical research to a minimum. The purposes of this book are to clearly define and explain adrenal fatigue, to provide tools to help you determine if you suffer from adrenal fatigue, and to deliver a concise course of action for you to achieve optimal health. The information presented is vastly superior to what most physicians know or understand. Please share it with those who are open-minded enough to learn.

A lot of thought went into the title of this book. I wanted it to grab your attention and to let you know that there is a solution to what you've been going through. My mission for this book is restoring your body's function and health. The original title, So Many Symptoms, fell short, because it was limited to treating symptoms.Misdiagnosed: The Adrenal Fatigue Link alerts the public to the fact that adrenal fatigue exists and is often misdiagnosed by physicians.

The cover of the book lists just a few of the misdiagnoses and symptoms associated with adrenal fatigue, but as you read on, you will discover many more. Adrenal fatigue was once just an incidental finding, but as life has become more stressful and non-stop, it has become epidemic. While this has been largely due to the changes in our lifestyle, equally significant are the failures of physicians to recognize the signs and symptoms of adrenal fatigue, to accept adrenal fatigue as a diagnosis, and to properly treat the patient.

To understand how adrenal fatigue occurs, let's take a look at the history. The adrenal glands were designed for a lifestyle that existed thousands of years ago and changed very little up until the twentieth century. The adrenal glands'main function was to help the body deal with imminent danger and stress. The adrenals are responsible for the fight-or-flight mechanism, which simply means that they give the body a short burst of adrenaline needed to either fight or run away from a dangerous or stressful situation. The adrenal glands are what give a mother the super-human strength to lift a car that has trapped her child underneath it or the energy to run away from a charging animal. By design, they are for short bursts of energy and long periods of rest. They were definitely not constructed for today's chronic and continuous physical and mental stress levels. Over two decades ago, when I began my practice, adrenal fatigue was a rarity, and I was finding only a few cases per year. Today, in my experience, it is a major diagnosis growing to pandemic proportions due to many contributing lifestyle factors, including high stress levels, poor diets, and lack of downtime, all compounded by the fact that adrenal fatigue symptoms vary greatly, and many sufferers have been misdiagnosed.

I first learned about the adrenal glands when I was in chiropractic school in the late 1980s. Like most physicians, my education was limited to the basics: the location of the adrenals, what nerve stimulates them, their blood flow, hormone production, and the diseases in which they may be involved. Traditional medical education on the adrenal glands does not mention adrenal fatigue, nor does it recognize that it even exists.

Traditional medicine believes that the adrenals can always meet your stress needs, unless they are diseased and become totally dysfunctional. The only times that diseases of the adrenal glands are accepted in traditional medicine are when the adrenals are totally broken and produce no hormones or are overstimulated due to either another chronic disease or cancer. Adrenal fatigue is not a diagnosis typically found in traditional medicine; it is a diagnosis adapted by functional medicine physicians to explain the dysfunction of the adrenal glands.

I did not fully appreciate the severity or complications relating to adrenal fatigue until I was working toward my certification in an advanced medical specialty called applied kinesiology. Applied kinesiology is as series of diagnostic and treatment protocols that work to optimize the body's performances on a physical, mental, and biochemical level. Applied kinesiologists recognize that the mind and body do not need to be diseased to manifest signs and symptoms, but that even minor dysfunction can cause health issues. (Dysfunction versus disease is a key point of this book; we need to correct dysfunctions in the mind and body in order to prevent diseases.) My introduction to applied kinesiology gave me the basic tools to recognize the signs and symptoms of adrenal fatigue as well as several basic treatment methods. While adrenal fatigue was emphasized, it was merely one of hundreds of special dysfunctions that could occur in mind and body. The true importance of adrenal fatigue treatment as the catalyst to good health would not be known to me for several more years.

During the first years of clinical practice, I was presented with a steep learning curve. I had to learn how to manage an office, my patients, and myself. I also had to determine how to effectively utilize the thousands of hours of academic knowledge I had acquired. It was during the first few years of clinical practice that I began to see how important and prevalent adrenal fatigue was in the general public. I quickly learned the difference between a life of academia and one spent in the real world.

Since chiropractic students practice on each other, they are learning from fellow students who are in their late twenties, extremely health-conscious, physically fit, and whose biggest worries revolve around schoolwork. The real world is filled with patients who are much older, care little about their health until it starts to wane, avoid physical exercise like the plague, and whose worries—family, work, and money—are much more intense. The difference between these two groups is so dramatic that what works on the academic group does not necessarily work on the general public. I quickly recognized that while both groups had physical aches and pains, the academic group's pains where from challenging their bodies with exercise, while the pains of the general public were from inactivity. I began to wonder: How could a group of people who barely challenge their joints, muscles, and tendons develop so many complaints? The reason became obvious when I started listening to my patients, who were talking less and less about their physical complaints and more and more about their personal lives and stressors. Instead of straining themselves with physical exercise, my patients were pushing their bodies to the limit with mental stress.

Early in my practice, I would mistakenly focus on the area of pain that the patient would complain most about. This mistake (focusing on the pain instead of the causes) was the way western medicine trained physicians to practice. It was not the way that eastern medicine trained physicians practice. I found that I was chasing the patients' pains around their bodies and often offering only temporary relief. This method of pain relief care became frustrating to the patient and to me. The situation was exacerbated by the fact that many patients were already mentally stressed and suffering with other conditions, like fatigue, poor sleep, and other systemic problems. I would often send for standard lab and diagnostic tests in an effort to find the underlying cause of their symptoms, but there would be no relevant findings. I began to ask myself some difficult questions.

Question: *How could a person have so many health issues and complaints but have no positive labs or diagnostic findings? What was I missing?*
Answer: I did not know!

Question: *How does the body deal with physical or mental stress?*
Answer: The fight-or-flight mechanism is activated for a short burst of energy utilizing the adrenal glands.

Question: *But this stress is chronic, so what if the adrenals could not handle the physical and mental stress load?*
Answer: The adrenals would become dysfunctional and adrenal fatigue would occur.

Then, I asked myself the original question again.

Question: *How could a person have so many health issues and complaints yet have no positive labs or diagnostic findings?*
Answer: Adrenal dysfunction leading to adrenal fatigue!

So, adrenal fatigue was the reason my patients had physical, emotional, and systemic complaints. Adrenal fatigue was the answer to why my patients felt mentally exhausted, had so many different aches and pains, had no positive lab findings, and responded poorly to traditional care. These patients were not suffering from multiple areas of pain, mental stress, and other systemic issues; they were suffering from one issue: adrenal fatigue. Adrenal fatigue was affecting my patients' energy levels, moods, and pain response. Adrenal fatigue was why they never felt a hundred percent relief. Correcting the adrenal fatigue was the answer to restoring my patients' health and vitality.

The realization that the average American experiences more mental stress then physical stress was a breakthrough for me and my patients. I immediately began to take the adrenal fatigue diagnostic protocols I had learned in my applied kinesiology training and use them during the initial evaluation of each patient. Those patients who tested positive for adrenal fatigue received treatment for their underlying adrenal dysfunction and for their pain symptoms. I quickly developed several additional tests to determine if my patients had adrenal fatigue and if they could handle the mental and physical stress they were encountering on a daily basis. My findings quickly showed that the average patient could barely handle the activities of their daily lives, let alone any additional stress or the healing process. Many patients would fall apart—physically or emotionally—with any additional stress or at the completion of a stressful situation. Evaluating my patients' ability to handle stress, and how that ability was linked to their adrenal response, was the key to healing my chronically ill, misdiagnosed, and most difficult patients.

In the late 1990s, adrenal fatigue took on a new level of importance in my practice. The 1990s were a go-go-go time in America. Nobody stopped. Times were good, and people were pushing themselves harder than ever. The popularity of the personal computer and cell phone made it easier for people to work, even at home and on weekends. The idea of the forty-hour work week was gone, and there was no time left for rest. People where burning themselves out at an unprecedented rate and were turning first to caffeine, and later to medications, to keep themselves going. The first signs of the adrenal fatigue epidemic were beginning to show.

This go-go-go approach to life, and to the adrenal fatigue that followed, led to a new disease called chronic fatigue syndrome (CFS). Just like adrenal fatigue, CFS had no positive lab or diagnostic findings but was diagnosed by the patient's history and physical complaints. CFS mirrored adrenal fatigue exactly. I concluded that CFS occurs when the adrenals cannot produce enough energy to keep a person energized. Chronic fatigue was the symptom, and adrenal fatigue was the underlying cause. CFS was the first signal that Americans were becoming overloaded and that adrenal fatigue was moving from an obscure finding to a major health issue affecting many Americans.

Chronic fatigue syndrome was quickly followed by the fibromyalgia epidemic. Fibromyalgia also mimicked adrenal fatigue in that it had no specific lab or diagnostic test but was diagnosed by the patient's history and vague physical exam. Fibromyalgia was the epitome of adrenal fatigue, because it had the same physical and emotional findings as advanced adrenal fatigue cases. I found that fibromyalgia patients had worn down their adrenal functions to the bear minimum, so, like CFS patients, they had no energy, but they also suffered with anxiety, depression, and chronic transient pain. Fibromyalgia sufferers had lost the ability to produce sufficient levels of several key hormones and neurotransmitters that the adrenal glands produce. Adrenal fatigue was not even being considered or recognized by most physicians and was already morphing into a more severe version of itself. I could already see the healthcare crisis on the horizon.

The stock market crashes in 2000 and 2008, the terrorist attacks on September 11, 2001, and the decades-long wars in the Middle East have resulted in an overwhelming amount of mental and physical fatigue. These events have led to a full-blown healthcare crisis focused on anxiety and depression, but the underlying adrenal fatigue has once again been ignored. The traditional treatments of antidepressants and anti-anxiety medications have led to a more than five-hundred-percent increase in their use in the United States in just the last ten years. It is estimated that one in four Americans takes an antidepressant or anti-anxiety medication on a daily basis.

These medications may help patients temporarily, but they do nothing to support the weakened adrenals. Medications merely enable the patient to continue on and thus weaken the adrenals even further. The delay caused by being misdiagnosed and treated with medications is now resulting in adrenal fatigue cases that are more severe, more difficult to treat, and are occurring in younger patients.

Adrenal fatigue has gone from an incidental finding in practice to an epidemic. The inability of modern medicine to recognize the signs and symptoms, along with the dramatic changes in our lifestyles, have led to this healthcare crisis. While fifteen years ago, the average age of a person in my office suffering with adrenal fatigue was between forty and fifty, I am now seeing severe cases in fourteen- to sixteen-year-olds. If we are to control and reverse the effects of this healthcare crisis, we must first understand adrenal fatigue's causes, symptoms, and treatments.

My goals for this book are to make the general public—and thus traditional physicians—aware that adrenal fatigue exists, to promote awareness in physicians that diagnostic lab tests are available to determine if adrenal fatigue is an issue, and most importantly, to let you, the reader, know that there is an answer to why you don't feel right. You may need to journey beyond basic medicine, but the results will be worth the trip.

A Doctor's Story

The Clear Choice

Every doctor has a story. There has to be a reason why we do what we do. For me, it was a very practical reason, initially.

When I was in high school, I developed migraines. The migraines were so severe that I would be completely incapacitated for two to three days a week. This would continue for weeks on end. No matter how many physicians my parents brought me to, I received no relief at all. Then one day my father, who suffered from chronic low back pain, mentioned my situation to his chiropractor.

"Let me try to help him," was the response my father got.

This was a long time ago, and although chiropractic had not yet evolved into what it is now, my migraines improved through the chiropractic care I received. They didn't totally disappear, however they did dissipate enough that I was able to go to college.

When it came time to make a choice about my career path, the decision was clear. I wasn't looking for a job that would have me sitting behind a desk; I wanted a career in which I would be actively adding quality and value to people's lives. As a good student, I had plenty of options. I had been planning on going to medical school, and for a long time, I thought I would be a neurosurgeon.

I remember thinking to myself: *I went to so many other physicians and got so little relief, or no relief, and then this simple chiropractor was able to give me substantial relief. I'm going to head into that career.*

Chiropractic School

So, in September of 1986, I began chiropractic school. This one event changed not only my life but the lives of a great many others, from the physicians I later taught (and all of their patients) to the thousands of patients I later treated.

When I was going through chiropractic school, there was huge diversity among the students. Some were only interested in adjusting the spine and taking care of muscle aches, neck pain, and back pain. I, on the other hand, saw the opportunity to explore how the mind and body work as one. I was not satisfied by dealing only with nerve impingement (which is extremely important and what chiropractic care excels at); I wanted to learn how the body interacts in a biochemical, emotional, and physical relationship. This led me to get involved in applied kinesiology.

Applied Kinesiology

In the United States, applied kinesiology is an offshoot of chiropractic, but throughout the world, it's a medical specialty,like orthopedic surgery, neurology, and cardiology. The benefit of applied kinesiology is that it allows the body to tell the physician where there is dysfunction. The basis for diagnosing and treating with applied kinesiology is to use muscle testing to determine if there are any of the following: nerve interference, an issue within the acupuncture meridians, blood flow issues, joint dysfunction, emotional stress, and any other issues that could impede proper brain and body function. Since this method of diagnosing and treating is based on what the body and mind are indicating, proper treatment always benefits the patient. Applied kinesiology, in conjunction with traditional exams and lab testing, gives the physician a more complete picture of why a patient has a health complaint and how best to proceed with treatment.

Applied kinesiology can help in the diagnosis of a physical problem, an emotional problem, a nutritional problem, or what I've found to be most common — a combination of all three. An example of a combined issue would be a person suffering from headaches that are caused by muscle tension in their neck from working long hours, and the long hours at work are achieved by drinking a lot of coffee. Since this person's complaint has an emotional, physical, and biochemical component, proper care and relief will only be achieved if all three components are addressed.

Armed with this new knowledge, I started taking on more ambiguous cases. While other chiropractors were dealing only with neck and back pain cases, I was working with more difficult and chronic cases, including migraines, temporomandibular joint (TMJ) pains, herniated discs, and gastrointestinal problems. My practice evolved into a clinic known for taking on the most challenging cases.

Clinical Nutrition

I continued my education to become a Certified Nutritional Specialist (one of only four hundred in the United States), a Diplomate in Nutrition (one of only three hundred in the United States), and a leader in combining nutrition with physical medicine. I found that the more I worked at this, the more enigmatic cases I received, and it became increasingly harder to achieve the desired results that my patients deserved. I began to discover a missing link in my care. This aspect — the one at which I was weakest — was addressing the emotional component of a health issue. I realized that if I wanted my patients to truly be healthy, I needed to explore new ways to help them deal with their depression, stress, and anxiety.

Neuro Emotional Technique

With the help of Dr. Howard Cohn, who wrote a chapter in this book about the health benefits of an alkaline diet, I discovered a technique called Neuro Emotional Technique (NET). NET uses visualization, acupressure points, and nutrition to help people overcome the effects of traumatic and stressful events that have been holding them back from being truly healthy. A person might have a terrible low back pain, mostly from a herniated disc, but also because they've experienced a great deal of emotional trauma and stress in their life. Emotional stress and trauma can get trapped in the nervous system and muscles and cause muscle pain, GI distress, and other symptoms. A simple example of this is when your neck or back gets tight when you have to visit your in-laws or talk to your boss. The best way to treat this type of condition is to use chiropractic care to relieve the physical pain, nutrition to relieve the inflammation and reduce the patient's stress level, and NET to release the emotional stress being held in the targeted area.

The Missing Link

By focusing on the mind and body aspect of my patients' health conditions, I was able to improve the outcome of their care, and more and more difficult cases began to arrive at my office. I found that the majority of patients were coming to my office focusing less on their physical pain; they were dealing with a lot of emotional and much more complex problems. These more intricate and emotional cases all seemed to have a common pattern; there seemed to be a weakness in one particular part of the body. The weakness that was continually showing up in these difficult cases was in the adrenal glands (the glands that sit on top of the kidneys). The adrenal glands were becoming fatigued, and when the adrenals became fatigued, my patients would develop much more difficult cases that involved both a physical and an emotional component.

As time went on, I found that when I addressed the adrenal fatigue problem, patients would respond faster and recover more fully. Even the most difficult cases would begin the healing process and would now respond positively to the adjunct therapies they were receiving. My experience in dealing with these complex cases challenged me to develop new techniques and methods to determine which patients had adrenal fatigue and the best way to care for them.

Years of experience and success have led me to be able to share some of the basics of what I learned, so that you can now determine if you have adrenal fatigue and how to start the healing process. While no book is a substitute for a good physician, it is a great place to start.

While you read this book, try to keep the following sentence in the front of your mind: Adrenal fatigue is not an emotional or physical issue but *a physiological dysfunction that affects you both physically and emotionally.*This simple sentence explains why adrenal fatigue is so difficult to diagnose and how it causes so many different health issues. Fortunately, it also makes adrenal fatigue very treatable and responsive to care.

If It Worked For The Marines, It Can Work For You!

I recently completed a research project designed to test the effectiveness of my adrenal fatigue protocols on the most difficult cases: combat exhausted Marines. I chose this group to test because they are the most difficult to treat in terms of the extent of their adrenal fatigue, location, and lifestyles, and because they are the most deserving of care. The United States military is overwhelmed with adrenal fatigue, or what is more commonly referred to as post-traumatic stress disorder (PTSD). The following is an abstract of my research project, which successfully treated burnout/resiliency/PTSD in Marines. The full study is being submitted in early 2014 for publication in medical journals.

Key points of the study:

- During the ninety-day study, 90 percent of Marines showed improvement

- No lifestyle changes (diet, combat, location, exercise, etc.) were made

- Physical and emotional complaints dropped by 40 to 50 percent in ninety days

- No negative side effects were noted

- Improvement was achieved by nutritional supplements alone; no other factors were involved

- Marines were tested and treated remotely; no personal contact with the physician was needed

This study was so successful that the treatment protocols are being reviewed by the Soldier On Foundation, the Wounded Warrior Project (WWP), the Veterans Health Administration, and the Pentagon for expansion as a primary treatment for soldiers, sailors, and Marines. If my program worked on combat exhausted Marines, it can work on you!

Topic: An Effective Nutritional Program to Treat Burnout/ Resiliency/PTSD in Military Personnel

Steven Zodkoy, DC, CNS, DCBCN, DACBN

Abstract: Burnout in military personnel has been well studied and documented, but a successful and viable treatment protocol has not been established. This article will review the results of a viable nutritional supplementation program to treat burnout and the associated conditions of resiliency and PTSD. PTSD is estimated to account for 20 to 39 percent of all cases seen by the Veterans Health Administration and to affect 12 to 19 percent of service personnel returning from deployment. While research has shown a link between burnout, resiliency, PTSD, and the biochemistry of the body, none of the military's present treatment strategies have successfully addressed these issues. Present treatment protocols for burnout, resiliency, and PTSD include: maintaining physical exercise, finding meaning and purpose in work, practicing religion and spirituality, developing coping skills, sustaining social support, practicing mind-body techniques, taking medications, practicing sound sleep routines, and utilizing cognitive behavioral therapy. Clinical lab testing of hormones and neurotransmitters has already been proven to be a reliable indicator for an increased risk of burnout, resiliency, and/or PTSD. This study demonstrates how nutritional supplementation, based on clinical lab testing, improves burnout scores by 41 percent (original Maslach Burnout Inventory [MBI] questionnaire mean score of -13.13 and a ninety-day MBI questionnaire score of 0.88). The results were significant upon evaluation by the Wilcoxon signed-rank test at $p<0.01$. Two participants (12.5 percent) achieved a "no burnout" status, while another two participants (12.5 percent) achieved a burnout ranking of "mild" upon completion of the program. This program has the added benefits of being deployable, expandable, and a having high compliancy rate, all of which are necessary to be effective for military implementation.

Lisa

Before going to Dr. Zodkoy, my fourteen-year-old daughter was very fatigued, had headaches, dizziness, joint and back pain, and even had heart palpitations. She was tired all the time and was going to bed around 7:00 PM. She was struggling to get through the day and had to stop playing on her school softball team.

I was looking into different specialists when I heard about Dr. Zodkoy. My daughter had gone through two rounds of blood work that tested for all different things. Each time, the doctor would call and say, "Good news! Your daughter doesn't have mono!" But it wasn't good news. I wanted to know what was wrong with her. She was tested for mononucleosis, diabetes, and Lyme disease. I thought she had a thyroid problem and asked the doctor for that test as well. But they all came up negative.

I was about to take her to the Philadelphia Children's Hospital when I decided to take my friend's advice and go to Dr. Zodkoy. When they told me about him, I felt better just hearing it.

She's now been seeing Dr. Zodkoy for about six weeks and is on all different supplements, including vitamins, minerals, probiotics, adrenal support, and lysine. It was gradual, but after five weeks, she was 75 percent better. At that point, Dr. Zodkoy was not happy with her progress, so he tested her again and found a virus in her system. Now she's doing much better. After six weeks of treatment, my daughter has started staying up later and is playing on her softball team again. Now, the fatigue she feels is from her busy schedule.

Chapter One
Do You Have Adrenal Fatigue?

Questionnaires

Determining if you have adrenal fatigue has as much to do with your history and how you feel as it does with lab tests and exam findings. The reason a patient's history and complaints are so important is because signs and symptoms of adrenal fatigue occur only when the body cannot meet the stress needs put on it by emotional, physical, and biochemical factors. These stress overloads occur much earlier than findings on lab tests. A physical exam—by a trained healthcare provider with experience in treating adrenal fatigue—is a great way to determine if you have adrenal fatigue, but finding someone qualified to help you can be difficult.

Questionnaires for adrenal fatigue and its earlier onset, burnout, have been utilized for decades with extreme accuracy. I use the Maslach Burnout Inventory (MBI) in my practice to measure how patients around the world are doing and for my work with military personnel with post-traumatic stress disorder (PTSD). The MBI is extremely useful for measuring emotional response to life and work. It has the added benefit of being correlated to cortisol production, a major hormone produced by the adrenal glands, and thus adrenal fatigue. The use of questionnaires to document and even diagnose adrenal fatigue is well accepted and is both time and cost efficient.

Volume and Variety of Complaints

The questionnaire is designed to take into account that many people have comorbidities: a primary health complaint and multiple secondary complaints.

One of the easiest ways to diagnose adrenal fatigue sufferers is by the number of physical, emotional, and general complaints they have. The sheer volume and variety of their complaints clearly indicates that a weakness in their core system, and not numerous separate problems, is causing the majority of their issue. While a typical patient may score high on a few select issues, adrenal fatigue sufferers usually score high in the emotional, physical, and general health areas.

It is important to remember and understand that not every sign and symptom of an adrenal fatigue sufferer has to be linked to adrenal fatigue. More likely, eighty to ninety percent of them are linked to adrenal fatigue, and the other ten to twenty percent are linked to aspects of everyday life that we all experience. It is possible to have a low back condition or allergies and also have adrenal fatigue, and the good news is that when you begin the lifestyle changes and nutritional program to treat adrenal fatigue, you will also help the body heal other ailments.

Self-Diagnosis

Adrenal fatigue is one of the few medical conditions that you can diagnose and then correct on your own. Because there are so few physicians aware of adrenal fatigue, after following the steps outlined in this book,self-diagnosis of adrenal fatigue is most likely what you'll be doing. I believe that nearly all cases of adrenal fatigue can be diagnosed by just listening to a patient's story and symptoms. The questions that follow are very similar to what I would be asking you if you were my patient. The score you derive at the end is just like me giving you a diagnosis at the end of a consult.

These questions reveal the most common complaints of adrenal fatigue sufferers. Adrenal fatigue hits each person differently, so it does not matter if you do not have every symptom or fit the mold exactly. Here are some of the statements commonly made by adrenal fatigue sufferers who do not want to admit there is a problem:

"Everyone has aches and pains."

"It is just my age."

"Everyone would score high on this test."

"Who doesn't have...?"

"It's genetic."

If you find yourself saying any of the above to yourself, you probably have adrenal fatigue. All of the above statements are true to an extent, but you have to realize that not everyone has as numerous and varied complaints as an adrenal fatigue sufferer. Not everyone feels so weak, achy, and desperate for an answer that they are reading this book.

The truth is that while healthy individuals may score high on a few select questions, adrenal fatigue sufferers tend to score high all over the test. If you have a bad back, you may have pain and need medications, but you should not have emotional issues or pain in other places. If you are clinically depressed, you may test poorly on those questions and need medications, but you shouldn't have anxiety, pain, sleep issues, or fatigue unless adrenal fatigue is a secondary issue. Adrenal fatigue is not just about the severity of your individual complaints but rather how vast and varied they are.

When completing the questionnaire, do not think about your answers; go with your gut. There are enough questions, and they are designed to make sure that the overall score is correct, even if a few answers are ambiguous. If you are unsure about what the question is asking, just answer it the way you think it should be answered. I have found that adrenal fatigue sufferers score far above the minimum acceptable number.

General Questions Linked to Adrenal Fatigue

1. Have you suffered an emotional trauma that you feel still affects you (examples: death, divorce, abuse, violence)?   YES NO

2. Have you suffered a physical trauma that you feel still affects you (examples: surgery, infection, accident)?
                                                        YES NO

3. Do you feel you have excessive anxiety or stress?
                                                        YES NO

4. Do you take or have you taken medication or supplements for anxiety or stress?   YES NO

5. Do you feel depressed, sad, or down?   YES NO

6. Do you take or have you taken medication for depression?   YES NO

7. Do you take or have you taken pain medication for more than two weeks?   YES NO

8. Do you treat or have you treated with a therapist, counselor, or psychiatrist?   YES NO

9. Have you seen multiple physicians for a single complaint? YES NO

10. Have you experienced a long period of stress (examples: school, family, work)? YES NO

11. Do you feel misdiagnosed? YES NO

12. Do you often feel misunderstood? YES NO

13. Have you ever been diagnosed with a chronic illness (examples: MS, hypothyroidism, heart disease, fibromyalgia, IBS, diabetes)? YES NO

14. Do you "just not feel right?" YES NO

15. Do you or did you have medical complaints but no positive lab findings (meaning you were not diagnosed with a disease)? YES NO

16. Have you been treated for a medical condition but have not responded to care? YES NO

17. Have you been to more than three doctors in the last two years? YES NO

18. Have you changed your lifestyle to avoid pain or anxiety (examples: given up a sport you enjoy or stopped attending a meeting)? YES NO

19. Do you or others think you're a hypochondriac? YES NO

20. Has your health put your life on hold? YES NO

General Question Total Score
(total number of YES answers multiplied by 3): _____
(maximum score is 60)

These general questions are worth more points, because they are about your core. These questions are about issues that, even when you are healed from adrenal fatigue, will still be factors and stressors in your life. This section gives a good indication of the extent to which your adrenal glands have been burdened on a physical and emotional level.

Physical Symptoms Linked to Adrenal Fatigue

Many patients develop adrenal fatigue after a traumatic physical event, such as a sports injury, car accident, fall, or explosion (I treat a lot of service personnel and veterans for whom this is a common occurrence). The physical injuries sustained in those events may seem to skew this section, but this section should be completed anyway. I have found that unless the traumatic event was truly extensive, the human body will heal itself. Often, the limiting factor in this healing process is not the extent of one's injuries; it is the fact that the adrenals are so fatigued after the trauma that they cannot support the healing process.

Physical trauma requires the adrenal glands to fight inflammation, produce energy, control anxiety, and more. Someone who has borderline adrenal dysfunction is often sent over the edge by a traumatic physical event into full blown adrenal fatigue. In this situation, the event is seen as the problem, and the adrenals are ignored. Since the adrenals are never strengthened, the person is never able to fully heal. I see this in military personnel with traumatic brain injuries (TBIs) from explosions, teens with sports injuries, and in the general public with all types of traumas. The best medical care cannot help these types of patients, because only the physical aspect of their problem is being addressed. Supporting their adrenal fatigue, in conjunction with other types of care, provides great relief.

Before completing the next set of questions, take a moment with the diagram below, placing an X on the areas in which you have had pain or a health problem in the last twenty-four months.

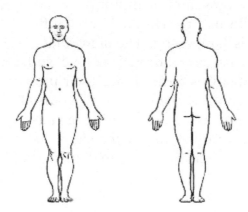

Total number of X's: _____. Typically, a person aged thirty to thirty-five will have 1, a person aged thirty-five to forty-five will have 2, and a person aged forty-five to fifty-five will have 3.

At this point, you may be asking yourself: *How can I have so many more physical complaints in so many different areas when the average person only has a couple?*
Answer: There must be a core problem causing the issues.

The physical signs and symptoms of adrenal fatigue are vast and vary greatly from person to person. The reason for this variety is that the adrenals control the nervous system and the endocrine (hormone secretion) system. The adrenals are involved in nearly every action the mind and body perform. The physical signs and symptoms that may occur with adrenal fatigue vary greatly with each adrenal fatigue sufferer, since they depend on the individual's genetics and lifestyle. For example, a data-entry worker with adrenal fatigue may have wrist pain, headaches, and neck pain (the areas under the most stress from their job), while a home keeper may notice more dizziness when picking up items around the house, or fatigue from climbing the stairs all day.

The physical signs and symptoms of adrenal fatigue are opportunistic in nature. They will attack the body where the most activity is happening. The signs and symptoms change so frequently, because adrenal fatigue sufferers adapt and change their lifestyles to minimize their problems. A key sign of adrenal fatigue is when you find yourself changing your normal patterns to avoid aggravating or causing pain. The vast variety and systemic nature of the signs and symptoms from which a person suffers is the key to diagnosing adrenal fatigue.

Use this scale to answer the following questions:

0 — not an issue

1 — mild problem in either severity or frequency (one time or less per week — barely notice the problem)

2 — moderate problem in either severity or frequency (two to three times per week — notice the issue, but it passes quickly without special care)

3 — severe problem in either degree or frequency (three or more times per week — issue requires care, such as rest, over-the-counter drugs, or prescription medication)

Physical Symptoms (score 0–3):

1. Headaches   —

2. Fatigue, even after resting   —

3. Neck pain   —

4. Lightheadedness or dizziness when walking or moving your head around ___

5. Dizziness upon rising from a bed or chair ___

6. Trigger points (muscle knots) ___

7. Muscle aches ___

8. Joint inflammation ___

9. Arthritis ___

10. Gastrointestinal issues (diarrhea or constipation) ___

11. Tendonitis ___

12. Bursitis ___

13. Migraines ___

14. Tension ___

15. Muscle fatigue ___

16. Low endurance ___

17. Low libido ___

18. Generalized pain ___

19. Fibromyalgia ___

20. Urination frequency ___

21. Excessive weight gain ___

22. Having chest or back pain that is worsened by a deep breath ___

23. Feeling more pain the day after exercise or physical labor ___

24. Joints feeling loose ___

25. Feeling better wearing a brace or support   __

26. Hurting during or after a massage   __

27. Awakening with pain that eases a little as the day goes on   __

28. Tending to have more energy later in the day   __

List all other physical complaints you have had in the last twelve months:

_____

_____

_____

_____

_____

_____

_____

Physical Symptom Total Score: __   (maximum score is 87)

Emotional Symptoms Linked to Adrenal Fatigue

The emotional part of the questionnaire seems to be the most difficult for people to complete. I think everyone wants to avoid being looked at as a downer or complainer, or as someone with psychological issues. The beauty of doing the questionnaire in this book is that you can be honest with yourself, and no one needs to know.

It may also help you to keep in mind that adrenal fatigue is a physiological problem that may be causing emotional issues; it is not a psychological issue. Modern medicine's failure to accept adrenal fatigue as a true disease has led to millions of Americans being misdiagnosed with psychological issues such as anxiety, depression, PTSD, and burnout. While many adrenal fatigue sufferers do not want to admit to themselves or to others that they are having emotional issues, it can be a lot easier to accept emotional issues when you realize that they are coming from a physical weakness and are not a mental illness. You wouldn't be upset if you felt weak and had strange thoughts due to being dehydrated, so why be upset when the depletion is not water but neurotransmitters or hormones from the adrenal glands?

As you go through the following questions, do not think about your answers. If you take more than ten seconds to decide on an answer, it is a YES.

Use this scale to answer the following questions:

0 — not an issue

1 — mild problem in either severity or frequency (one time or less per week — barely notice the problem)

2 — moderate problem in either severity or frequency (two to three times per week — notice the issue, but it passes quickly without special care)

3 — severe problem in either degree or frequency (three or more times per week — issue requires care, such as rest, over-the-counter drugs, or prescription medication)

Emotional Symptoms (score 0–3):

1. Do you feel hopelessness or despair?   ___

2. Do people irritate you when driving or standing in line?   ___

3. Has your tolerance for everyone and everything decreased?   ___

4. Are you less productive at home and work?   ___

5. Do you have unexplained fears and anxieties?   ___

6. Do you feel unwell often?   ___

7. Do you find it difficult to deal with any type of stress?   ___

8. Do you try to avoid people, sometimes even friends and family?   ___

9. Do you feel depressed?   ___

10. Do you feel burned out?   ___

11. Do you prefer to be alone?   ___

12. Do you have anger?   ___

13. Do you have low self-esteem?   ___

14. Do you feel grief?   ___

15. Do you feel paralyzed in life?   ___

16. Do you have resentment?   ___

17. Do you feel unemotional, detached, or lacking in positive emotions?   ___

18. Do you feel dread or paranoia?   ___

19. Do you feel compelled to neatness? ___

20. Have you become obsessive (or more obsessive)? ___

21. Have you lost the sense of joy? ___

22. Do you have insomnia one or more times per week? (If you take anything to help you sleep, mark YES) ___

23. Have you lost the lust for life? ___

24. Has sex become a chore? ___

25. Have you thought of hurting yourself? ___

Emotional Symptom Total Score: _____ (maximum score is 75)

Lifestyle Questions Linked to Adrenal Fatigue

Negative Lifestyle Questions:

1. Do you smoke?   YES NO

2. Do you do illegal drugs?   YES NO

3. Do you have three or more alcoholic drinks per week?
   YES NO

4. Do you drink coffee (decaf included)?   YES NO

5. Do you eat less than three vegetables per day?
   YES NO

6. Do you eat less than three fruits per day?   YES NO

7. Do you sleep less than seven to eight hours per night?
   YES NO

8. Do you commute more than half an hour to work each way?   YES NO

9. Do you sit most of the day?　　　　　YES　NO

10. Are you overweight?　　　　　YES　NO

11. Do you drink soda or ice tea (diet, low-calorie, and decaf included)?　　　　　YES　NO

12. Do you drink energy drinks?　　　　　YES　NO

13. Do you eat at fast food restaurants?　　　　　YES　NO

Negative Lifestyle Total Score (total number of YES answers multiplied by 5): _____ (maximum score is 65)

Positive Lifestyle Questions:

1. Do you exercise three or more times per week?
    　　　　　YES　NO

2. Do you eat fruits three or more times per day?
    　　　　　YES　NO

3. Do you eat vegetables three or more times per day?
    　　　　　YES　NO

4. Do you take vitamins?　　　　　YES　NO

5. Do you get seven to eight hours of sleep per night?
    　　　　　YES　NO

6. Do you drink forty-eight ounces of plain water per day?　　　　　YES　NO

7. Do you have a caring family that you engage with (talk, dine, play games) a few quality times per week?
    　　　　　YES　NO

8. Do you have friends to socialize with (talk, dine, play games) a few quality times per week?　　YES　NO

9. Do you have a pet?   YES NO

10. Do you have activities you enjoy doing?   YES NO

11. Do you regularly read for entertainment?   YES NO

12. Do you take time for yourself during the week?
                                                             YES NO

13. Do you try to put yourself first sometimes? YES NO

Positive Lifestyle Total Score (total number of YES answers multiplied by 5): _____ (maximum score is 65)

Add the following:

General Questions Score: _____ (out of 60)

Physical Symptoms Score: _____ (out of 87)

Emotional Symptoms Score: _____ (out of 75)

Negative Lifestyle Score: _____ (out of 65)

Subtract:

Positive Lifestyle Score: _____ (out of 65)

Total score: _____

What does your score mean?

A score of 20 or above is a clear indication of adrenal fatigue, and the higher your score, the more severe your condition. I would advise that rather than concentrating on your score or the severity of your condition, just focus on the fact that you have adrenal fatigue. The simple facts are: you are either healthy, or you are not healthy; you either have adrenal fatigue, or you do not have adrenal fatigue. The severity of your condition does not matter; only the fact that you need to improve your health matters. The steps for a severe adrenal fatigue case and a mild case are the same; the only difference is how long it will take to rebuild your health. The majority of adrenal fatigue cases begin to respond within weeks of lifestyle changes and nutritional support. Severe cases make a more dramatic improvement in the beginning and are often more motivated to continue the healing process.

You have the most immediate control over your lifestyle habits, both positive and negative, and you can exercise that control right now by reviewing how you answered those sections above and beginning to work on improving your scores in those sections. If you scored poorly on the positive lifestyle points, stop reading and go get a vegetable snack. *Go!* The lifestyle sections are so important, because they show you that you have control over your condition, and that you can begin to make positive changes right away. Every time you make a good decision on the positive lifestyle list, you are heading for good health and happiness; every poor decision moves you closer to pain and unhappiness. You cannot have a negative lifestyle and expect to be happy and healthy.

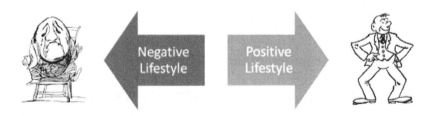

I recommend that you retake this test every thirty days to monitor your improvement. If a particular area of complaints does not improve, make sure you get a consult from a health care professional, as it may indicate a problem not related to adrenal fatigue. You can adapt your nutritional supplements dosage and treatment as your score improves. The lifestyle habits you adopt to improve your health should continue for life—a long and healthy life.

Ellen

For a long time, I was experiencing debilitating migraines. They were so terrible that I was non-functioning. I could not keep up with my daily activities and found no relief in any medications.

I went to a doctor who diagnosed me with occipital neuralgia. Still, nothing worked to relieve my migraines.

Then I went to Dr. Zodkoy. He diagnosed me with adrenal fatigue and started me on adrenal cortex supplements. I felt better within two weeks.

When I stopped the adrenal cortex supplement, without consulting Dr. Zodkoy, my migraines returned immediately. I now take my adrenal cortex supplement religiously, and I am feeling a hundred percent better.

Chapter Two
What is Adrenal Fatigue?

"Adrenal fatigue is used to describe the adrenal glands' loss of proper hormonal regulation in response to chronic physical and/or emotional stress."
— Dr. Steven Zodkoy

Adrenal Dysfunction

The term "adrenal fatigue" is commonly used to describe what happens to the adrenal glands when they cannot keep up with the physical and emotional stress the body is experiencing. Adrenal fatigue is used as the diagnostic term for the condition, because it is both descriptive and easy to understand, but a better term would be adrenal dysfunction. Adrenal dysfunction better illustrates the process of how the adrenal glands overreact or fail to react over time to continued stress. The adrenal glands do not just fail; they first become fatigued and reduce their activity over time. There are several steps in the process of becoming adrenal fatigued, and often the first and second steps involve the adrenals overproducing hormones. Adrenal dysfunction is a more accurate name for this condition, because it better describes how the adrenals no longer properly respond to stress, and it better accounts for the overproduction of some hormones and the underproduction of others. Adrenal fatigue is the end stage of adrenal dysfunction. Since this is precisely when most patients experience the most severe symptoms and begin seeking help, let's stick with the term adrenal fatigue for our purposes.

How Does Adrenal Fatigue Occur?

Your adrenal glands are designed to respond to acute stress and then subsequently relax. Today's world is filled with dozens of perpetual, low-grade stressors that constantly keep the adrenals functioning at a slightly heightened level. Mobile phones, computers, email, an ever-increasing number of television channels, careers, and relationships are all on twenty-four/ seven and therefore all require a response from the adrenals. Compare today's world to the one of just fifty years ago, when life was much slower and time off was time off. There were no mobile phones, no computers, only three television channels, one family phone line, no terrorist threats, and fewer "crazies" in the United States—all of which allowed for downtime and for the adrenals to turn off. Compare that life to the one of two hundred or ten thousand years prior, when people rose and slept by the sun, and the pace of life was unimaginably slower. The past was filled with plenty of downtime—time for the adrenals to rebuild themselves. While the world has advanced to become a twenty-four/seven potpourri of stimulants, the human body's response to the stimulus has not advanced since the Stone Age. The loss of true downtime in the modern world has led to the proliferation of adrenal fatigue.

Adrenal fatigue rarely happens all at once but is rather a gradual and steady decline in the adrenals' ability to respond to stress. Most people with adrenal fatigue will state that they have felt emotional or physical stress for a long time. Examples of physical stress include working long hours, chronic illness, and lack of downtime. Examples of emotional stress include school, work, family, an abusive relationship, illness, depression, and anxiety. These chronic stressors set the stage for adrenal fatigue.

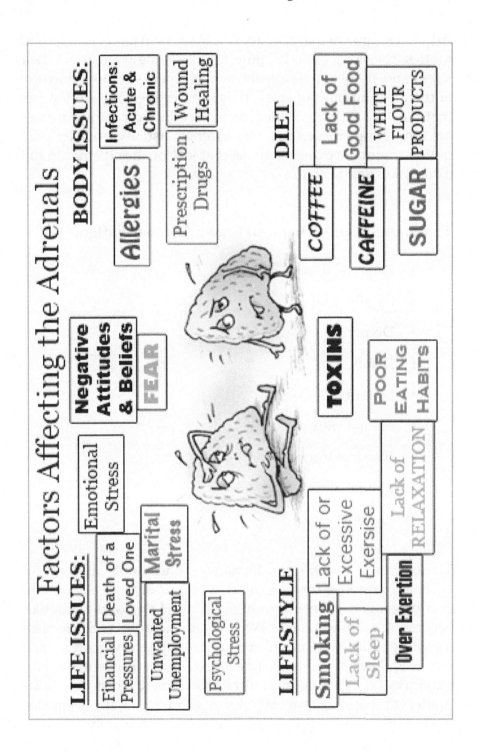

Factors Affecting the Adrenals

LIFE ISSUES:

Financial Pressures
Death of a Loved One
Emotional Stress
Unwanted Unemployment
Marital Stress
Psychological Stress

Negative Attitudes & Beliefs
FEAR

BODY ISSUES:

Infections: Acute & Chronic
Allergies
Prescription Drugs
Wound Healing

DIET

COFFEE
CAFFEINE
Lack of Good Food
WHITE FLOUR PRODUCTS
SUGAR

LIFESTYLE

Smoking
Lack of or Excessive Exersise
Lack of Sleep
Over Exertion
Lack of RELAXATION
TOXINS
POOR EATING HABITS

Adrenal fatigue usually occurs when a person has been exposed to stress for a long period of time. Many people are aware of their stress and its negative impact, while others—although aware of the great amount of stress they are experiencing—often feel that they are thriving under stress. In either case, the adrenals are struggling to keep up. The adrenals usually do keep pace until a traumatic event happens that just pushes them into full exhaustion and fatigue.

Traumatic Events That Can Cause Adrenal Fatigue

- Personal illness

- Family illness

- Divorce

- Death

- Loss of job

- Mental trauma

- Physical trauma

- Mental abuse

- Physical abuse

These events require production of enormous amounts of adrenal hormones for an extended period of time. At the end of a prolonged exposure to high levels of stress, the adrenals become totally fatigued. While some people with adrenal fatigue will have a long history of feeling overwhelmed, and others will only experience one acute traumatic event, the vast majority of adrenal fatigue sufferers will have a history of low-grade, chronic stress followed by an acute traumatic event that pushes them over the edge. The relationship between how the body and mind respond to stress was best explained by Professor Robert M. Yerkes in 1908.

Yerkes-Dodson Law Explains Adrenal Fatigue

The Yerkes-Dodson law (see Figure 1) was developed to explain the relationship between stress and how the body performs. It was originally developed by Robert M. Yerkes and John Dillingham Dodson in 1908 but has since been adapted by numerous other researchers. The first part of the law states that performance increases — and can be maintained — with low-level physical or mental stress. It explains how we are regularly able to handle the simple stressors of school, work, and family (represented by the dotted line in Figure 1). The second part of the law states that performance increases with complicated or overwhelming stress, but only up to a point. When the stress levels become too high, performance begins to decrease rapidly. It explains how we start to lose productivity when our lives become overwhelmed with longer work days, long commutes, financial problems, and family difficulties, and how we can at first meet the challenges but later often feel overwhelmed by them if they continue for too long (represented by the solid line in Figure 1). It also explains why traumatic events overwhelm our adrenals and can cause our health to decline quickly. These two parts are represented in the graph below.

Image of the Yerkes-Dodson Law

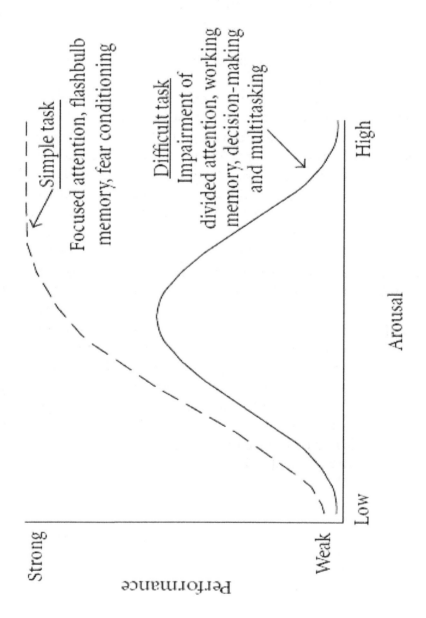

Figure 1

The most common presentation of the Yerkes-Dodson law is represented by Professor Donald O. Hebb's graph (Figure 2), which omits the representation of low-level stress that does not affect the performance of simple tasks (represented by the dotted line in Figure 1). The Hebbian process is often illustrated graphically as an inverted U-shaped curve that increases and then decreases with higher levels of arousal (Figure 2). The Yerkes-Dodson law and Hebbian graph are excellent representations of what happens to the adrenals when they are overstimulated by stress. The first half of the graph shows how the body will adapt to stress by increasing function and response. The second half of the graph shows how the adrenal function and ability to cope drops as the stress continues.

Hebbian Graph of the Human Performance Curve

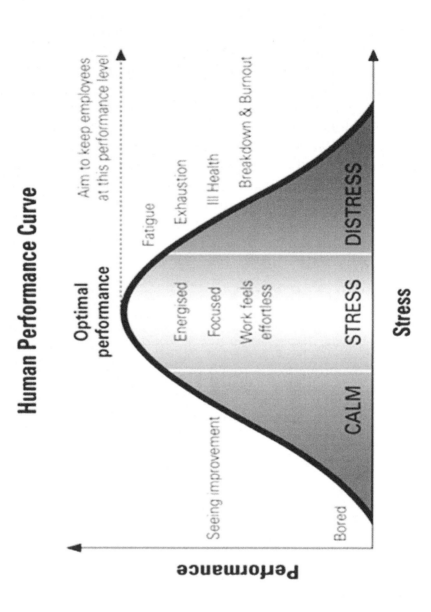

Figure 2

The Yerkes-Dodson law explains why at the beginning of a stressful situation, people often feel strong and alert. A person then reaches a point at which they cannot take any more, and they start to develop symptoms. The Hebbian graph can also represent the adrenals'output during that time. They are at first able to produce large quantities of hormones to meet the needs caused by the stress, but then they reach a point of exhaustion and begin to decline. Health symptoms begin to appear when the adrenals can no longer balance the stress levels of the mind and body.

The Hebbian graph can also help explain why adrenal fatigue is so difficult to diagnose with conventional lab tests. A single lab reading of the adrenal hormones would likely give an adequate—maybe even high—reading on either side of the optimal point, as illustrated by points A and F on Figure 3, but the physiological and emotional difference between points A and F are dramatic. At point A, the person feels good and is handling their stress; at point F, they have already reached their breaking point and are experiencing signs and symptoms of adrenal fatigue. So even though points A and F have the same lab results, the patient feels completely different. It is this and other quirks in lab testing that make adrenal fatigue difficult to diagnose.

The fact that the same lab test reading can mean two different things makes both conventional lab testing and conventional medicine obsolete in diagnosing adrenal fatigue. Understanding the three stages of adrenal fatigue will also help you to grasp why it is so often misdiagnosed by traditional medicine. While conventional lab testing may be inadequate to test for adrenal fatigue, there are several lab tests that are suitable, and these will be explained in later chapters.

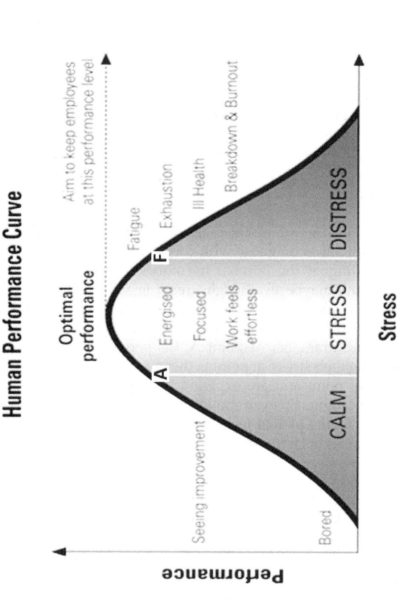

Figure 3

Early-Stage Adrenal Fatigue

The early stage of adrenal fatigue is a sweet spot for many sufferers, and it can last for decades or just a few weeks depending upon genetics, overall health, and past experiences with stress. Before the early stage, a person may have some physical and emotional complaints, but for the most part, they are getting through life on an even keel. This stage is engaged as the person's stress level starts to increase and overwhelm their normal coping mechanisms.

During the early stage, a person usually feels great. They know they are under stress, but they feel that they are performing well and handling or even thriving under the extra stress. This is due to the adrenal glands initiating the fight-or-flight mechanism and thus flooding the body with hormones and neurotransmitters to deal with stress. The fight-or-flight mechanism is an all-or-nothing response, so at the beginning, the hormonal release from the adrenal glands greatly out paces the body's needs. Due to the abundance of adrenal hormones in the early stage, there are usually few or no physical or mental complaints. This sense of well-being often lulls the person into complacency about the effects of long-term stress, and they take few, if any, actions to limit and mediate the causes of their stress. At this point,the adrenals are ready for action and have plenty of reserves to endure stress. The adrenal glands do not have to choose between the production of dehydroepiandrosterone (DHEA), cortisol, epinephrine, norepinephrine or serotonin, because they are strong enough to produce them all. A person in the early stage of adrenal fatigue is usually feeling good, but it isn't a healthy good. This stage is the equivalent of being in shock after an acute event. The body is producing so many hormones that physical and mental problems are hidden. When those hormones start to reduce, the onset of physical and mental symptoms is swift and dramatic.

The following is what happens to hormones and neurotransmitters produced by the adrenals in the early stage of adrenal fatigue:

> Cortisol is being produced at a very high level in the early stage of adrenal fatigue. At first, high cortisol will reduce inflammation and provide plenty of energy for the body by increasing glucose levels in the blood. The extra cortisol makes the person feel minimal pain and energized. Serotonin levels are optimized at this stage. Serotonin is utilized by the nervous system and the brain to promote a sense of calm and well-being. This person may realize that they are under stress, but may feel like they are thriving under it. They have energy but also a sense of calm about them. DHEA is also being produced at adequate levels. DHEA is the precursor to testosterone, estrogen, progesterone, and other key hormones. The ready availability of these key hormones adds to the sense of well-being. Often, women will find that their menstrual cycle improves during this stage. Epinephrine (adrenaline) and norepinephrine are important hormones and neurotransmitters for the nervous system. Their high levels at this stage give a person a sense of keen mental alertness. Physically, the extra epinephrine makes a person feel strong and powerful.

The early stage of adrenal fatigue is earmarked by how well the patient feels and is responding to stress. This sense of well-being is misleading and is present at the cost of exhausting the reserves and the future ability of the adrenals to deal with stressors. Unfortunately, Americans are trained to be concerned about their health only when they are experiencing pain and symptoms. The lack of concern over the stress a person feels and its damaging effects is not an effective way to deal with stressors, and it almost always leads the person into the next stage of adrenal fatigue.

The duration of the early stage of adrenal fatigue—the sense of well-being or thriving under stress—varies greatly in people. I have treated young children who are already experiencing adrenal fatigue from problems during their birth or due to childhood abuse. On the other hand, I have found retiring military officers who experienced decades of combat and are perfectly fine. A person's ability to maintain this stage has a lot to do with their genetics, coping mechanisms, and environment. If a person in the early stage of adrenal fatigue does not get rest or find a way to mitigate their stress, they will eventually use up all their hormone reserves, thereby reducing the ability of the adrenals to deal with stress. As the stress continues and the adrenals' reserves are depleted, problems and symptoms will start to appear. The heightened sense of well-being associated with this early stage will quickly fade, only to make the later stages of adrenal fatigue that much worse.

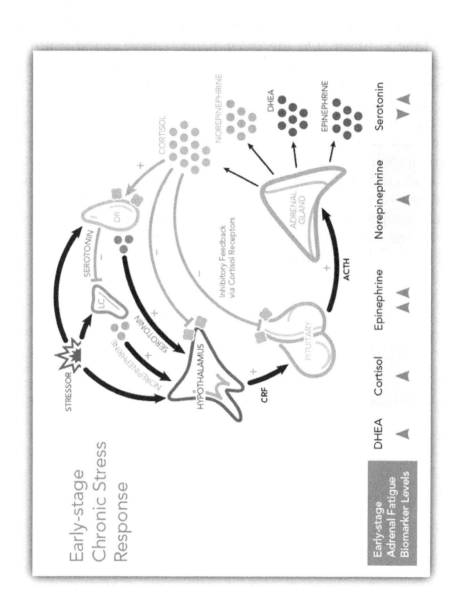

Mid-Stage Adrenal Fatigue

The adrenals can handle chronic or acute stress for only so long before beginning to waiver. Mid stage in the adrenal fatigue process is when a person starts to succumb to their stress, and the adrenals begin to give out. There is no exact moment or event that marks the point when a person's stress starts to outpace the adrenals'ability to maintain balance. The earmarks of this stage are when physical and/or emotional symptoms begin to show, the sense of well-being disappears, and a person no longer feels that they are handling their stress as well as they have in the past. The mid stage of adrenal fatigue is usually the point when a person realizes something is not right, but it is not necessarily when they seek help or try to change their lifestyle. This is the stage of false hope, when a person believes that their physical and emotional symptoms will pass on their own. People in this stage are counting on a vacation or for life to slow down for a quick recovery.

The mid stage of adrenal fatigue is when the adrenal glands try to prioritize the hormonal needs of the body and then match their production. By this stage in adrenal fatigue, the hormonal reserves are depleted, and all hormonal needs from the adrenals must be met by immediate production. The problem with having no hormonal reserves is that demand always outpaces production. When demand exceeds production, the only solution the adrenal glands have is to prioritize which hormones are needed most and should be produced at any given moment. This prioritizing of hormonal demand always leaves a deficiency somewhere. The prioritizing of hormone production is akin to paying the past-due electric bill while letting the water and gas bills go unpaid. Eventually, you have to pay a larger water and gas bill, and the deficit will grow. When hormone productions are insufficient or vacillating, physical and emotional symptoms really start to show.

During mid-stage adrenal fatigue, DHEA, cortisol, epinephrine, and norepinephrine may be found to be high or low depending upon the immediate stress and need of the body. DHEA may be high during a woman's menstrual cycle but then quickly drop well below normal once it passes. Epinephrine may shoot up in a risky situation but drop below safe levels the rest of the time, causing symptoms like fatigue, asthma, or pain. The low periods and the swing in hormones during this stage are what cause signs and symptoms of adrenal fatigue to begin to show. A key marker found in the mid stage of adrenal fatigue is that serotonin levels drop. Serotonin is a major hormone in the body and neurotransmitter in the brain. Low levels of serotonin in the body have been associated with pain, restless leg syndrome, fibromyalgia, and other pain syndromes. Low levels of serotonin in the brain that are associated with depression are often treated with medications called selective serotonin reuptake inhibitors (SSRIs), which include medications such as Paxil® (paroxetine), Zoloft® (sertraline), and Celexa® (citalopram). Serotonin is the first hormone to decline in adrenal fatigue, and that alone can cause serious physical and emotional symptoms to develop.

The symptoms that start to arise during mid-stage adrenal fatigue start off slowly and mildly. The low-grade symptoms of this stage often do not stimulate a person to action. The personmay feel that a little rest and relaxation will restore their health, and they may not realize the extent of the damage their mind and body are undergoing.

The end of mid-stage adrenal fatigue is usually when the first misdiagnosis occurs. Toward the end of the mid stage, the symptoms of adrenal fatigue begin to become undeniable. Fatigue, mood changes, anxiety, aches and pains, and loss of desire are noticeable enough that a medical consult is scheduled. Depending on the type of physician seen and what the major complaint of the day is for the patient, this almost always results in a misdiagnosis. Common misdiagnoses at this stage are anxiety, depression, "just aging,"premenopausal, fibromyalgia, low testosterone, psychosomatic illness, generalized pain, cluster headaches, migraines, and just about every other diagnosis available. Medications are usually prescribed at this time and often offer some relief for the one symptom they are designed to help, but other symptoms worsen, and more complaints arise.

Mid-stage adrenal fatigue often ends with a patient knowing that they do not feel right but being misdiagnosed on what is causing the problem. During this stage, they still hope that a little rest or a slow-down in their fast-paced life will remedy the problem. Since proper care was not received and no lifestyle changes were made, the adrenal fatigue continues to worsen and develops into end-stage adrenal fatigue.

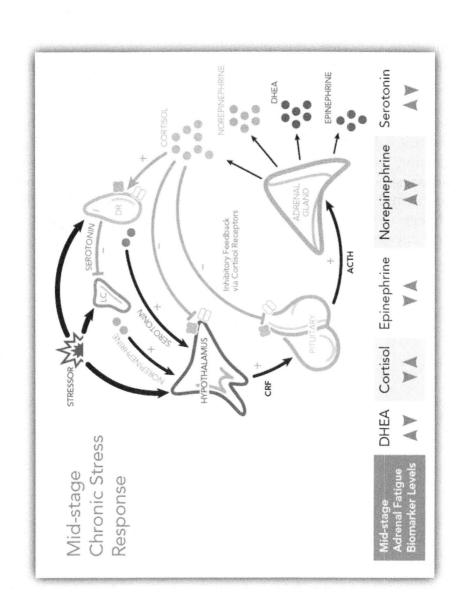

End-Stage Adrenal Fatigue

The end stage of adrenal fatigue is the easiest to recognize and write about. People in the end stage of adrenal fatigue have undeniable physical and/or emotional symptoms. It is no longer a question of *if* something is wrong but rather of *what* is wrong. This stage is highlighted by the numerous unexplained complaints, and the sufferers are forced to alter their daily routine just to get through the day. During this stage, the symptoms are irrefutable, and often additional medical consults are scheduled. Countless medical tests are ordered, different medications are tried, and copious misdiagnoses are given. Often, the medications tried offer limited and temporary relief to one of the symptoms, but it is quickly realized that the majority of the symptoms are still present. Frustration and fear are the hallmarks of the end stage of adrenal fatigue. Sufferers are forced to seek alternative care and diagnoses because of the undeniable deterioration of their health.

I most often see patients at the end stage of adrenal fatigue, presenting with a myriad of symptoms and complaints. Their medical records are thick with lab testing, x-rays, MRIs, and medical consults, with no concrete diagnosis. They are often on several medications and taking numerous nutritional supplements—sometimes self-prescribed—in an effort to restore their health. This is when antidepressants and anti-anxiety medication are pushed on them by their physicians— another misdiagnosis that only allows the adrenal fatigue to worsen. Their physicians and family members often believe that the underlying problem is all emotional, but the patient knows that there is something more to their condition.

During the end stage of adrenal fatigue, the adrenals cannot produce enough cortisol, DHEA, norepinephrine, epinephrine, or serotonin. The patient usually has numerous emotional and physical complaints. Common statements given by patients are,

"I am falling apart,""I am going crazy,"and "I am not myself."In this stage, adrenal hormone production is so compromised that any physical or emotional stress is met with a new round of symptoms and complaints. The simple tasks of daily living become a series of huge chores and the quality of life declines.

Unfortunately, many sufferers go months, years, or even their entire lifetime without receiving the right diagnosis or care. As their health deteriorates, so does their personal life. Their interest in friends and hobbies disappears. Relationships with family members become strained, as they cannot participate in life's events. Often they become solitary or withdrawn and develop emotional issues. End-stage adrenal fatigue sufferers spend their lives in a vicious pattern of doctor visits, misdiagnoses, and medications. There are a lucky few who find their way to proper care with a physician skilled in diagnosing and treating adrenal fatigue. These lucky few have their lives restored, almost like magic, as proper care for their adrenal fatigue is started. Adrenal fatigue is one of the few serious health conditions that can be reversed with proper care.

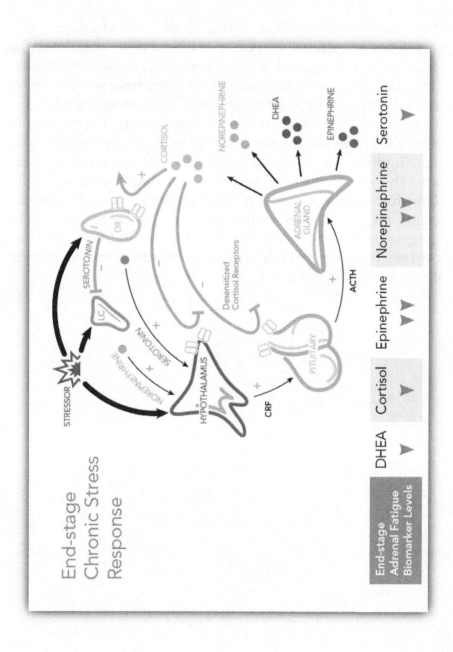

Patient Response to Proper Care

There are several amazing things about adrenal fatigue. The prevalence of adrenal fatigue in the American population is remarkable. I estimate that 25 percent of those over the age of forty, and 50 percent of those over age fifty, have some stage of adrenal fatigue. The severity and variations of adrenal fatigue are numerous in scope; no other condition can affect a person in so many different emotional and physical ways. But the most amazing thing about adrenal fatigue is how well it responds to care. The worst and most severe cases of adrenal fatigue will begin to respond within weeks of proper care, and dramatic results are often seen within months. The human body is designed to heal from even the most severe conditions, and the recovery from adrenal fatigue is a great example of the body's ability to rebuild and move on.

Laura

Before going to Dr. Zodkoy, I never felt right. I suffered with many symptoms, including depression, fatigue, muscle aches, and anxiety. I was also waking up throughout the night, which made me feel even more fatigued on a daily basis. Everyday activities became a challenge, and I could not function as normal.

I began to see a therapist for the depression, because everyday life was unbearable. When the symptoms became too difficult, I went in search of an antidepressant.

When I still had no relief, I went to a physician to have blood work done in the hope that something would come up that could explain why I was feeling off. Nothing came back conclusive.

At that point, I went to Dr. Zodkoy's office. He diagnosed me with adrenal fatigue and put me on many different supplements. It was as if I went from 0 percent to 80 percent overnight. My physical pain went down dramatically, and everyday activities were possible. I could tackle problems in a calm manner, because I wasn't so anxious and worrying all the time.

I have been following Dr. Zodkoy's regimen for three months now, and I feel 95 to 98 percent better. I could not be happier that I went to Dr. Zodkoy. He made me feel normal again.

Chapter Three
What are the Adrenals Glands and What Do They Do?

The Big Picture

Because the adrenal glands are responsible for so many physical and emotional actions, adrenal fatigue can be very difficult to understand, but with a little background information, the general concept can easily be understood. The goal of this book is not to educate you on the complex interactions of the adrenal glands, but to introduce you to this often overlooked and extremely important problem. When reading this chapter, try to focus on the big picture surrounding adrenal fatigue. Do not worry about remembering what each hormone does or trying to figure out which hormone is dysfunctional in your case. Instead, accept that the adrenal glands perform a myriad of complex functions and that any disruption will cause you both physical and emotional symptoms. If you can grasp the concept that the adrenal glands are an integral part of how we feel — and that even a minor change in their function has dramatic effects on our health — then you will have a better understanding of how the adrenals work than do most physicians.

Major Endocrine Glands
Male   Female

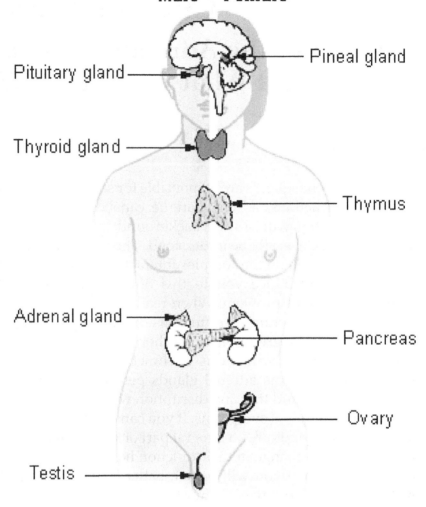

The adrenal glands are located atop each of the kidneys and have a combined weight of about ten grams in an adult. They are part of the endocrine system, which means they secrete hormones in order to affect how the body functions, and are most commonly associated with how the body deals with stress. The fight-or-flight response mechanism is controlled by the adrenal glands. It refers to the dramatic increase in adrenaline and other hormones necessary to engage with or run away from a threatening event. The adrenals are unique in that each adrenal gland has two distinct and autonomous parts. The outer part is known as the adrenal cortex, and the inner part is known as the adrenal medulla. While both parts of the adrenal glands produce hormones, their similarities stop there. Each part produces different hormones, acts independently of the other, is stimulated differently than the other, and is responsible for different reactions in the body.

The Adrenal Cortex

The adrenal cortex is devoted to production of corticosteroids and androgenic hormones. It is stimulated into action by hormones released from the pituitary gland, which is found in the brain. The fact that the adrenal cortex is controlled by the brain is the key to the mind-body relationship. This link between the mind and body is why most people with adrenal fatigue have both physical and emotional complaints. It is also why when we correct the physical weakness in the adrenals, patients' emotional complaints also disappear.

The adrenal cortex produces corticosteroids which are involved in a wide range of physiological processes. Having the proper amount of corticosteroids is key to a healthy stress response, immune response, inflammatory response, carbohydrate metabolism, protein catabolism, healthy blood electrolyte levels, and healthy behavior. Even a minor dysfunction in the response from the adrenal cortex would give you symptoms, including anxiety, agitation, insomnia, depression, pain, dizziness, fatigue, or weakness. The adrenal cortex produces three types of hormones: glucocorticoids, mineralocorticoids, and androgens.

Cortisol

The major glucocorticoid hormone produced by the adrenal cortex is cortisol. It is released in response to physical, emotional, or biochemical stress. Its primary functions are to increase blood sugar, suppress the immune system, and aid metabolism, all of which prepare the body to deal with stress more effectively.

Cortisol increases the blood sugar level via gluconeogenesis and glycogenolysis, both of which occur in the liver. Gluconeogenesis is a process in which the liver turns small proteins, called amino acids, into glucose. Glycogenolysis is the process in which the liver breaks down a complex sugar molecule, known as glycogen, into glucose. The goal of both of these processes is to give the body as much energy as possible for maximal brain function and body response to overcome the stress that triggered the response.

Cortisol also plays a significant role in suppressing the body's immune responses, which are the biochemical pathways that cause inflammation. The capability to reduce inflammation has made cortisol's derivatives—hydrocortisone cream, prednisone, and cortisone—a major tool in modern medicine. Hydrocortisone cream is sold over the counter to treat rashes, bug bites, and itchiness. Prednisone is a very powerful prescription drug used to reduce systemic swelling from ailments, such as arthritis and poison oak. Cortisone is used as an injection to treat severe tendonitis and bursitis.

Cortisol and Memory

A major new finding is how cortisol affects memory. A short burst of cortisol has been shown to help create a useful memory. Long-term exposure to cortisol in a stressful situation has been shown to be the cause of negative memories being trapped in our minds. There is also evidence that these trapped memories cause all other memories to be dulled, so that the mind can only focus on the negative, trapped memory. This cortisol-induced trapped memory is thought to be the mechanism for causing PTSD.

Cortisol's Other Effects:

- Counteracts insulin — raises glucose levels in the blood, leading to weight gain when the adrenals fatigue

- Reduces collagen formation, leading to joint and muscle pain when the adrenals fatigue

- Increases amino acids in blood

- Regulates sodium and potassium in blood to optimize pH

- Acts as an antidiuretic, leading to an increase in the frequency of urination when the adrenals fatigue

- Increases blood pressure due to vasoconstriction, leading to low or erratic blood pressure when the adrenals fatigue

- Causes temporary infertility

- Acts as antihistamine

- Stimulates liver detoxification

- Strengthens contractions of cardiac muscle

Normal Cortisol Production Pattern

Cortisol production varies throughout the day and night (see Cortisol Graph). Levels are highest in the morning and then decline by up to eighty percent by late evening. This pattern assures that we are energized in the morning and relaxed at night. Any change to the cortisol pattern can cause severe physical and emotional symptoms, including fatigue, anxiety, insomnia, and depression. The latest research on PTSD and depression has been linked to a flat diurnal (daily) cortisol pattern. In determining a correlation between cortisol and a particular health concern, a single sample is usually inadequate. One sample may be within normal range, but it is the daily cortisol level that determines proper function. To ensure proper adrenal function, several samples must be taken throughout the day. Unfortunately, most physicians only take a single sample, and this is precisely why patients go undiagnosed or are misdiagnosed.

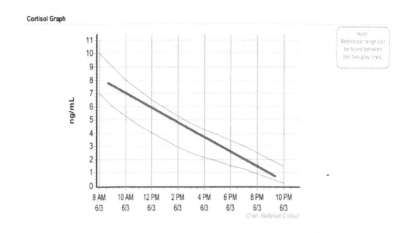

Normal Cortisol Production Throughout the Day

Aldosterone

The major mineralocorticoid produced by the adrenal cortex is aldosterone. Its main function is to reabsorb water through the large intestine in order to maintain proper blood volume and thus blood pressure. Aldosterone accomplishes this by reabsorbing sodium (and the water that follows) while releasing potassium through the intestinal wall. Aldosterone is a key to maintaining proper blood pressure and blood flow to the brain. Any disturbance to aldosterone functions can lead to dizziness, headaches, fainting, and confusion.

Androgens

The third set of hormones produced by the adrenal cortex are androgens, which are involved in the production of male hormones but are produced and necessary in women also. Androgens have been shown to directly affect certain brain functions and are linked to aggression and libido. The best known androgen hormone is testosterone, but there are several other important ones, including dihydrotestosterone (DHT), androstenedione (andro), and dehydroepiandrosterone (DHEA).

Testosterone has a variety of effects, the major one being the development of the secondary sexual characteristics in males. Testosterone is also important in building muscle mass, stimulating cell growth, maintaining a general sense of well-being, and generating sexual desire for both men and women. Low testosterone levels have been associated with muscle weakness, fatigue, low libido, and anxiety.

DHT is a more potent androgenic hormone that works similar to testosterone. Andro is converted to both testosterone and estrone and is critical to normal sexual function and the menstrual cycle. DHEA, a natural precursor to estrogen, is essential to normal female development, the menstrual cycle, and fertility. DHEA is of key importance in clinical practice, because low levels have been shown to be a precursor to PTSD and anxiety. Low levels of DHEA have presented in menopausal women experiencing hot flashes and are, therefore, pivotal in treatment.

Hot Topic: DHEA is derived directly from cholesterol. The over use of statins to lower cholesterol in adults in their twenties and thirties may be contributing to lower DHEA and hormone production and may lead to infertility.

The Adrenal Medulla

The adrenal medulla is the inner part of the adrenal glands. It is responsible for producing a hormone group called catecholamines, which include the following hormones: epinephrine (adrenaline), norepinephrine (noradrenaline), and a small amount of dopamine. These hormones have a major effect on the nervous system. In fact, they control the sympathetic part of the autonomic nervous system (ANS), which unconsciously runs the core of the body (all the things we do not think about). This is how we breathe, pump blood, urinate, become sexually aroused, digest, and maintain all the other bodily functions that take place without our control or input. The ANS has two parts: the sympathetic and the parasympathetic. The adrenal medulla hormones are the stimulating, or excitatory,hormones of the sympathetic ANS, and the parasympathetic part of the ANS is suppressing, or relaxing, in nature. The adrenal medulla hormones are not made in the adrenal glands. The adrenal medulla is stimulated into action by the nervous system, which has triggers and receptors throughout the body.

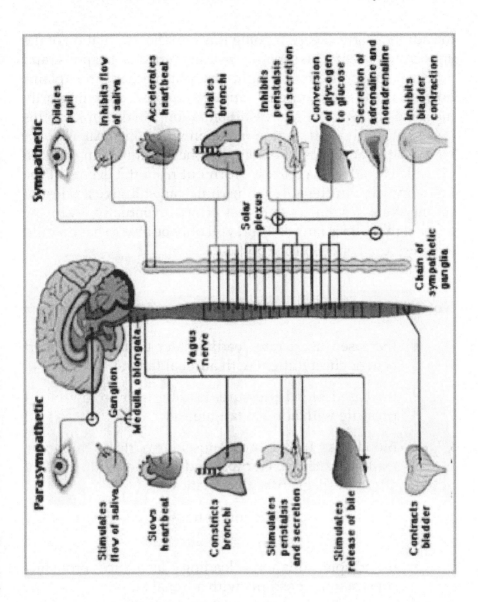

The epinephrine and norepinephrine hormones are primarily responsible for the fight-or-flight mechanism. Since these hormones work on the nervous system, they produce a much faster response than the hormones created by the adrenal cortex. The adrenal medulla initiates the fight-or-flight mechanism instantly through the stimulation of the nervous system, and the adrenal cortex keeps it going through the stimulation of the endocrine system. This separation of an immediate response and a delayed response to the fight-or-flight mechanism explains how even end-stage adrenal fatigue sufferers can temporarily meet the challenge of a stressful situation. An example of this is seen in nearly every action movie in which the beaten-down hero surges, at the last moment, to a new stimulus in order to prevail. The adrenal cortex is worn out from the events of the entire movie, but the adrenal medulla can still give a boost to the nervous system for one last effort. Eventually, even the adrenal medulla is fatigued and will only be able to have a mild and very brief effect on the body.

Notable Effects of Adrenal Medulla Hormones:

- Increased heart rate, leading later to an erratic heart beat or chest flutters with adrenal fatigue

- Increased blood pressure, leading later to low blood pressure with adrenal fatigue

- Blood vessel dilation to muscular parts of the body, leading later to cramps and fatigue with adrenal fatigue, especially with activities

- Blood vessel constriction to non-muscular parts of the body

- Bronchiole dilation, leading later to bronchial constriction or asthma with adrenal fatigue

- Increased metabolism, leading later to a slow metabolism and weight gain with adrenal fatigue

- Decreased GI function, leading later to constipation and/or diarrhea with adrenal fatigue

Epinephrine (adrenaline) is well known for its "magical"effects on the body. It is what gives a mother the strength to move a car to rescue her trapped child. It is given to asthma patients to open their bronchial passages and to those in anaphylactic shock (severe allergic reaction). The adrenal glands'ability to continuously produce this key hormone in the proper amount is nothing less than lifesaving.

The adrenal glands are not well suited for the over-stimulating modern world. The fight-or-flight mechanism was vital in prehistoric times, when there were threats all around. Today, this system is rarely used for true threats but is overstimulated by more chronic stressors, including phones, computers, work, and our modern lifestyle. It is these constant, low-grade stressors that are wearing down the fight-or-flight mechanism and the adrenal glands. The adrenal glands'inability to produce enough adrenaline when needed is a major cause of PTSD in the worst cases, and general anxiety in the less severe, more common cases. We are becoming a nation unable to deal with any stress, let alone a life crisis.

Think of it this way: Years ago, if our ancestors saw a lion, their stress levels spiked and their reaction was to prepare to fight or to turn and run like mad. Their adrenal glands made sure they had the energy and power to do either one of those short-burst activities. Today when we see a lion, we are more likely to try to get a good picture, because we are at the zoo. The adrenals are now pumping up to help you fight the stress of traffic, crowds, getting your child to smile for a photo, and the dead phone battery. Today's stressors are low-grade and chronic, giving very little time for the adrenal glands to rejuvenate.

Being the link between the mind and the body, the adrenal glands are therefore the link between life's stressors and the body. They were designed to be engaged for short bursts of energy, responding to acute and sudden stressors. They were not designed for today's modern world filled with chronic, low-grade stressors. Adrenal fatigue occurs because the adrenal glands were designed for an ancient time and have not evolved for today's lifestyle.

Melissa

For a long time, I had very debilitating symptoms that prevented me from accomplishing daily tasks. Most of all, I felt pure exhaustion. I had trouble falling asleep, and when I did, I would wake up in the morning feeling unrested. I never felt that I had a good night's sleep. This tiredness also made me moody, because I was so frustrated with feeling this way.I could not understand why I felt this way when I ate healthily and exercised often.

I went to my physician and had blood work done. The only thing that came up positive was for Epstein-Barr virus, and the doctors told me there was nothing I could do about it. Even so, the doctor also said that it shouldn't be making me feel the way I did. I had no energy or drive to get anything done that I wanted to do.

When I finally went to Dr. Zodkoy, he did a saliva and urine test on me. The results showed exactly what was wrong with me. It felt so good to finally have an answer. When I saw my results, I knew that it was not in my head.

I went on the supplements that Dr. Zodkoy gave me, and a month later, I had energy for the first time in a long time. It felt as if my body was being rebuilt. My energy levels were increasing and then so was my mood. The results also showed that my cortisol levels were so low in the morning and high at night, which explained my insomnia and tiredness in the morning. Dr. Zodkoy was able to develop a supplement regimen that would make my levels equal throughout the day.

After four to six weeks, I was markedly better. Then, in the follow up appointments, Dr. Zodkoy was able to adjust my herbs as necessary to keep me feeling my best.

Dr. Zodkoy understood my struggle and frustration. Others probably feel how I did — that they know something is wrong and can't find the answer. Dr. Zodkoy found the answer.

Chapter Four
So Many Symptoms
from One Problem

Pathology

When I was in chiropractic school, I took a class called pathology. Pathology is the study of diseases, teaching the signs and symptoms, the lab findings, and every minute detail of how a disease can ravage the body. My friend Eric L. was in the class with me, and every few weeks he would call me, stressed and worried that he had the disease being discussed that day in class. It didn't matter if the disease was found only in pregnant women in the southern hemisphere; without fail, he had it and was going to die. And the way he talked about it, his death was going to be at that very moment. Luckily, Eric survived every disease we learned about and now practices in Northern California. The purpose of this story is to help you realize two important things before reading on. First, even though adrenal fatigue can have severe and numerous symptoms, you most likely will not have them all or have them to the full extent. Second, adrenal fatigue is reversible, and most symptoms will all reverse once you start a rejuvenation regimen. Like Eric, you will survive and live a wonderful and productive life, better for knowing what adrenal fatigue is, what it can cause, and how best to treat it.

Adrenal Fatigue and Other Diseases

The purpose of this chapter is to show you how the symptoms of adrenal fatigue relate to other diseases, not to explain all aspects of the diseases or symptoms. If your health condition is not mentioned, it does not mean that the adrenals are not involved. If you scored high on the questionnaire section, your adrenals are fatigued and are involved in your health condition. To get an idea of how adrenal fatigue is affecting you, I suggest you read the sections that most closely resemble your condition.

The hormones produced by the adrenal glands are so important to every cell in our bodies, every moment of the day, that even the smallest imbalance or dysfunction can cause symptoms. These symptoms are often misdiagnosed as diseases. At the same time, adrenal fatigue is working behind the scenes in many common diagnoses, making the condition worse and slowing a patient's recovery. This chapter will explain how adrenal fatigue is often the real underlying issue with many of today's prevalent healthcare matters. While adrenal fatigue does not have to be the only cause of these symptoms, it is usually a key factor that needs to be addressed as part of the overall healing process.

When you read through this section, you will realize that there is a great deal of overlap. For example, PTSD and burnout are very similar except for the triggering event. They both involve multiple symptoms listed as separate issues. The overlap in symptoms and the similarity of different conditions just adds to the misdiagnosis of adrenal fatigue. A physician needs to focus on the possible causes of all these symptoms instead of just labeling each complaint with a separate diagnosis. American medicine is based on giving the "right" diagnosis so that the physician can get paid, not on giving the right diagnosis to heal the patient. Orthostatic hypotension is a billable diagnosis with a medication to correct it, so its treatment is payable by insurance companies. Adrenal fatigue is the most common cause of orthostatic hypertension, but since it is not an accepted diagnosis and is treated by nutritional supplements, it is not paid for by insurance companies. I provided the information in this chapter so that you can see how many diagnoses and symptoms found today are related to adrenal fatigue. I do not want you to match your symptoms to the diagnosis but rather to realize that the name of the diagnosis isn't important. Treating the adrenal fatigue that causes the symptoms which lead to the misdiagnosis is what matters most.

Burnout

When you feel that you are just going through the motions and have lost the joy and excitement of work or life, you may have burnout. Burnout can be thought of as PTSD minus the major traumatic event triggers. Burnout is found at the end stage of adrenal fatigue, when the adrenals are producing just enough hormones to keep you going but are not strong enough to produce a full response. The inability of the adrenals to fully respond to stressors makes a person feel dull or numb to their environment and later agitated and annoyed.

Symptoms of burnout are both physical and emotional in nature. The most common physical signs of burnout are dizziness, fatigue, and poor sleep. The most common emotional symptoms of burnout are anger, agitation, dull or numb feeling, loss of empathy, and depression.

Fibromyalgia

Fibromyalgia is a disease with a strong link between the mind and the body. Fibromyalgia sufferers have multiple physical and emotional symptoms that are all caused by adrenal fatigue. Typical physical complaints of fibromyalgia include fatigue, dizziness, inflammation, poor sleep, and muscle pains that move around the body. A typical fibromyalgia patient has a history of feeling stressed but also of feeling driven by the stress — one of those people who says, "stress motivated me" or "Ithrived on stress." Emotional symptoms include anxiety, confusion, depression, and nervousness. The physical complaints of fibromyalgia include muscle pains, joint pain, fatigue, dizziness, and "just not feeling right."

Typically, fibromyalgia occurs six to eighteen months after a physical or emotional trauma, such as a death, illness, divorce, or auto accident. The disease is triggered by the traumatic event, which causes the adrenal glands to burst into action to meet the hormonal needs brought on by the trauma. This overreaction by the adrenals causes them to become exhausted and speed through the stages of adrenal fatigue at a rapid pace. This is why fibromyalgia patients go from mild physical symptoms to full-blown physical and emotional symptoms very quickly. In these cases, the adrenals become fatigued more quickly than in others.

The adrenals are involved in fibromyalgia through the production of the hormones norepinephrine and epinephrine. These hormones are utilized by the body to control muscle contraction, blood flow, and inflammation. When their production is limited by adrenal fatigue, physical symptoms begin to occur. These hormones are also correlated to serotonin production in the brain. A reduction in serotonin can lead to anxiety, depression, and pain.

Cortisol levels are high in the early stages of adrenal fatigue, which helps a patient manage inflammation throughout the body. A high cortisol level has the negative effect of damaging and slowing the repair process of collagen found in skin, tendons, and ligaments. In fibromyalgia patients, this damage to the fibrous tissues of the body leads to pain, muscle weakness, inflammation, and even premature aging, causing patients to appear older from sagging and wrinkling of their skin. Collagen is fibrous rope that keeps the body held together. When it becomes weak the body just falls apart.

Medical physicians will often focus on the emotional symptoms of fibromyalgia by giving patients a selective serotonin reuptake inhibitor (SSRI) drug. This treatment will offer mild relief, but it does nothing to correct the adrenal fatigue or the physical aspect of the problem. Often, even more medications are used to treat the physical complaints.

Note of Interest: All fibromyalgia patients have very low saliva pH levels. An alkaline diet and nutritional support for adrenal fatigue will raise their pH. There is an inverse correlation between the saliva pH and the severity of their symptoms. As saliva pH levels rise, physical and emotional symptoms decrease.

Having treated thousands of fibromyalgia patients, I have found that the greatest difficulty is in getting them to believe that they can get better. Those who go on my programs for adrenal fatigue and alkaline diet do extremely well, experiencing an increased quality of life in just months. By tracking their saliva pH, I can tell when they are healed and when they are just in remission from their symptoms. I strongly suggest that anyone suffering from fibromyalgia have their saliva pH checked.

Post-Traumatic Stress Disorder

Treating post-traumatic stress disorder (PTSD) is a passion of mine. I first got involved in treating PTSD at the request of a United States Marine Corps general who wanted a solution for those in her command suffering from the disorder. Treating service personnel and civilians with PTSD has become a large part of my practice. The program I designed for the active personnel and veterans is now being reviewed for a national program that has the potential of helping tens of thousands.

The biochemistry of how adrenal fatigue is involved in PTSD — and, by extrapolation, the other conditions mentioned in this section — is very well studied. The epidemic of PTSD in the military has led to numerous research studies that show exactly how PTSD occurs in the brain. During a traumatic event, the body is producing large quantities of the adrenal hormones cortisol, norepinephrine, and epinephrine. The fight-or-flight mechanism is fully operational. Research now shows that large amounts of cortisol trap negative memories in the brain. When the traumatic event ends, the protective fight-or-flight hormones should drop and the production of the productive adrenal hormone DHEA should begin. It is the lack of the adrenal hormone DHEA following the traumatic event that leads to PTSD.

My research indicates that DHEA is not released in PTSD cases due to adrenal fatigue. The adrenal glands are so fatigued from supplying hormones to meet the needs of the traumatic event, and the needs of a lifetime of low-level stress, that when the time comes to produce the protective hormone DHEA, they are unable. Most PTSD sufferers are in the early or middle stage of adrenal fatigue, and the traumatic event sends them directly into end-stage adrenal fatigue. During end-stage adrenal fatigue, the adrenals are unable to produce adequate hormones to stabilize the body. This would explain why only some people get PTSD and why those in the military, with their twenty-four/seven lifestyle, have so many cases.

PTSD is not only restricted to military personnel. In the United States, the number one cause of PTSD is thought to be sexual abuse. Other causes of PTSD in the general public are auto accidents, traumas, financial crises, and witnessing traumatic events on television. PTSD can be caused by any real or perceived, firsthand or secondhand event that overwhelms the adrenal glands.

Dizziness, Light-Headedness, Orthostatic Hypotension, and Blood Pressure Problems

Orthostatic hypotension is a very common complaint with adrenal fatigue sufferers. It is caused by a sudden drop in blood pressure, leading to a temporary loss of blood flow to the brain. A person usually feels dizzy or light-headed when they arise from a seated or lying down position too quickly. There are several ways that adrenal fatigue is involved in this problem. The autonomic nervous system, which the adrenal glands control, is responsible for vascular constriction. The medulla area of the adrenal glands is responsible for the production of norepinephrine, which in turn is responsible for constricting blood vessels in order to maintain proper blood pressure at all times.

The early stages of adrenal fatigue usually cause an uptick in the production of norepinephrine, resulting in higher blood pressure. This may be detected by a physician, and medication will be prescribed to lower the blood pressure. When the end stage of adrenal fatigue is reached, norepinephrine levels drop, and there is less constriction of blood vessels, causing lower blood pressure. This situation could be compounded by the blood-pressure medications that were prescribed for the high blood pressure in the early stage of adrenal fatigue.

The cortex part of the adrenals produces the hormone aldosterone. This hormone works within the kidneys to reabsorb sodium, and consequently water, which leads to increased blood pressure. The early stages of adrenal fatigue may cause an uptick in this hormone and lead to slightly higher blood pressure. This may be detected by a physician, and medication will be prescribed to lower the blood pressure. When the end stage of adrenal fatigue occurs, aldosterone levels drop, less sodium and water are reabsorbed, and blood pressure drops. This situation may also be compounded by the blood pressure medication.

To further complicate the situation, the adrenal glands' first response to increased stress is to overproduce hormones, which causes increased vascular constriction and is a key part of the fight-or-flight mechanism. The body wants to keep the brain alert and ready, so it increases blood pressure via vascular constriction. The body's normal response to increased vasoconstriction is to increase serotonin, which is the primary method by which the body promotes vasodilation. Since serotonin relaxes the mind and body, chronic stress alsocauses increased serotonin production, causing additional blood vessel dilation. This all leads to a loss of control in the regulation of the blood vessels, blood pressure issues, and numerous other symptoms.

Heart Disease and Blood Pressure

There has been a lot of recent research on how the adrenal hormones are involved in cardiac events. High levels of the adrenal hormones cortisol and aldosterone have each been linked as an indicator for heart disease. Considering that most cardiac events are caused by a decrease in blood flow to the heart and that the adrenal hormones are responsible for controlling blood pressure and blood vessel constriction, research into this area needs to be explored. It is well known that stress and anxiety increases a person's risk for a cardiac event, and adrenal fatigue is the link.

Adrenal fatigue is all about losing control of the hormones produced by the adrenal glands. The adrenal hormones are involved with controlling blood pressure via water reabsorption, mineral reabsorption, and blood vessel constriction. A loss in regulation of adrenal hormones can lead to either low or high blood pressure — each capable of triggering a cardiac event.

Often with the adrenal glands, it is not overproduction or underproduction of hormones that causes problems; it is the loss of control. The adrenal hormones should normally stay within a consistent range. When the adrenals are fatigued, the hormone levels tend to move out of the normal ranges, and when they go too low or too high, they trigger a dramatic reversal. This dramatic reversal in hormone production is often what generates emotional and physical symptoms.

An Example: The adrenals are fatigued, so they are not producing enough hormones to maintain normal blood pressure. The blood pressure drops to critically low levels, and the person feels fatigued, weak, sweaty, and dizzy. The adrenals respond to this critical state by overproducing hormones in fight-or-flight manner, causing dramatic blood-vessel constriction and an increase in heart rate. The high blood pressure and heart rate can then easily turn into a cardiac event.

Fatigue, Insomnia, and Poor Sleep

The most common complaint in physicians' offices has to be fatigue. Fatigue accompanies almost every other disease and symptom mentioned in this chapter. The relationship between fatigue and the adrenals is obvious as well as subtle. The adrenals produce the hormones cortisol, norepinephrine, and epinephrine, which allow us to spring into action. Adrenal fatigue would reduce the production of these hormones and make a person feel fatigued and sluggish. When adrenal hormone production interferes with normal sleep patterns, the feeling of fatigue will become even more severe, often sending a person to bed for days at a time. This extreme fatigue is often misdiagnosed as depression, an infection, or anemia.

Insomnia is also a common sign of adrenal fatigue. A person suffering from adrenal fatigue often produces hormones at the wrong time, which is why a good cortisol test has to have four samples taken throughout the day. The adrenal-stimulating hormones secreted by the pituitary gland are usually greatest in the morning and taper off as the day goes on. Those with adrenal fatigue often have lab tests that show their adrenal production of stimulating hormones surging at the end of the day, making sleep difficult, which causes fatigue the next day. This type of person always describes themself as a night owl, having great difficulty getting up in the morning. What is actually happening to this person is that their adrenals are so fatigued, they cannot respond early in the morning.Because it takes them hours to get into full production, it is not until the actual time that the adrenal stimulating hormones should be tapering off that they are just getting started. Insomnia is given as the diagnosis, but adrenal fatigue is the problem. Medications taken to help with the insomnia do nothing to fix the underlying problem with the adrenal glands, so the condition worsens and maybe even develops into sleep apnea.

Anxiety and Depression

There have always been anxiety and depression sufferers but never to the extent that we have now in society. The greatest reason for the large increase in sufferers is linked to the changes in our lifestyle and the associated burden it puts on our minds and bodies. Our lifestyles have changed from a quiet life on the farm with plenty of downtime to a go-go-go routine of the city and suburbia. This dramatic change increase in lifestyle stressors has occurred in only the last hundred years, and we have failed to adapt as a society. This failure to adapt to our present lifestyle is probably the single largest cause of adrenal fatigue.

It is estimated that twenty percent of all Americans are on some form of anti-anxiety or anti-depressant medication. It is also widely accepted that less than half of those in need of help for anxiety or depression seek the care they need, which means that almost half of all Americans are suffering with either anxiety or depression. Research has shown that the vast majority of anxiety sufferers are truly adrenal fatigue sufferers who are misdiagnosed. The severity and likelihood of having depression has also been linked to adrenal fatigue. These misdiagnoses of anxiety and depression, which would be properly diagnosed as adrenal fatigue, explain why the medications used to treat these issues have such limited success. Research has often shown that prescription medication offers only a few percentage points greater relief than taking a placebo. The misdiagnoses of these conditions would explain why anxiety and depression are so rampant in our society.

Overproduction or underproduction of many of the adrenal hormones can cause anxiety. The early stage of adrenal fatigue is marked by the overproduction of the fight-or-flight hormones. Having too many excitatory hormones, when there is nothing to fight-or-flight away from, is a major reason for anxiety. Examples of the overproduction of adrenal hormones causing anxiety would be the nervousness before a speech or the overreaction to stress at home or work.

The underproduction of the adrenal hormones found in the late stage of adrenal fatigue can also cause anxiety. Low adrenal hormone production can lead to low blood sugar levels and decreased blood flow to the brain, both of which can cause anxiety. Often, it is the loss of control of the normal regulation of the adrenal glands that causes anxiety. When the adrenal glands become fatigued, they have a difficult time maintaining the normal balance of hormones in your system and often swing from one extreme to the other. Anxiety can occur when the adrenal glands go from producing too many hormones to producing very few hormones or vice versa. The dramatic swing in the production hormones is a major cause of anxiety.

Research has shown that many cases of depression are linked to adrenal fatigue by several different pathways. A person's inability to deal with life's stressors due to adrenal fatigue can cause depression. The adrenal glands' inability to produce enough DHEA to help cleanse negative memories can also lead to depression. The general malaise, pain, and fatigue often associated with adrenal fatigue are enough to depress anyone. In all of these scenarios, depression is a symptom, not the disease.

Addictions

I have treated thousands of people with all types of addictions — from gambling, to smoking, to alcohol and drugs — and in every case, there was an adrenal fatigue issue. It is difficult to say which came first, addiction or adrenal fatigue, but what is clear is that without addressing the adrenal fatigue, the road to recovery often fails and is much more difficult. Addictions are used as an artificial stimulus to force the adrenals to over produce hormones, producing a euphoric effect for the addict. The failure of physicians to recognize the link between adrenal fatigue and addiction has led to millions of ruined lives.

Recent research has linked many addictions to cortisol levels and other adrenal hormones. The easiest example to explain this interaction is gambling addiction. A person with a gambling addiction and adrenal fatigue is looking for a way to raise their excitatory hormones. Remember, most people with end-stage adrenal fatigue are "numb" or don't feel regular emotions. The excitement of placing a bet, win or lose, stimulates the fight-or-flight mechanism, causing their adrenal hormones to surge and allowing them to feel emotions. This same mechanism could explain adrenaline junkies and sex addicts.

Smoking cigarettes has been shown to raise cortisol levels and keep them high. This high cortisol, coupled with raised dopamine levels from smoking, is a very addictive combination. High cortisol and dopamine levels give a person the feeling of well-being, and that feeling is addictive. Quitting smoking causes both cortisol and dopamine levels to drop and dramatically adds to the difficulty of breaking the addiction.

Addicts of all types need to have their adrenal glands supported with nutritional supplements. Proper nutritional supplementation will help keep an addict's adrenal production at a sufficient level, so that they may begin to heal. While adrenal fatigue is not the only part of the addiction problem, if it is not addressed, it can be an unnecessary major hurdle for the addict to overcome.

Anger and Frustration

I have linked anger and frustration together, because prolonged frustration leads to anger. It is well documented that high adrenal hormone levels are present when a person is angry. This is the "fight" part of the fight-or-flight mechanism. The same process also works in reverse when high levels of adrenal hormones makes a person agitated, frustrated, and angry. This is what happens to a person is in the early stage of adrenal fatigue. During the early stage of adrenal fatigue, the adrenals are overcompensating for the stress they are under by pumping out high levels of adrenal hormones. These high levels of hormones often cause an agitated feeling and prime a person for a fight or confrontation. This scenario is similar to a bodybuilder on steroids—"roided out" and ready for a fight— except that the steroids are coming from the adrenal glands and not a medication.

During the later stages of adrenal fatigue, a person is much more frustrated because of their inability to function due to the lower adrenal hormone levels. A quick and effective way to force the body to produce more hormones is to go from frustration to anger, triggering the fight-or-flight mechanism. This process is done subconsciously and is often perceived as a person losing control. If the stimulus is enough (and anger is a great stimulus),the adrenal glands can almost always respond with a burst of very short energy.

Depression

I covered anxiety and depression together earlier in this chapter, because they often go hand in hand. There are also a number of cases in which the sufferer has depressiononly and no anxiety,and I wanted to make sure that those sufferers had a section to themselves. Depression is such a major problem in our society and so poorly understood that any program offering some promise of help should be fully explored.

It is estimated that up to twenty percent of all Americans suffer with depression and that only eight percent are on medication. The comorbidity between depression and adrenal fatigue is extremely high. Adrenal fatigue may not always be the direct cause of depression but almost always makes it impossible for a person to handle or recover from it. Depression is physically and emotionally draining, which puts a huge strain on the adrenal glands and lowers their production. The reduced adrenal hormone production makes it more difficult to deal with the depression, and so it becomes more severe and chronic, creating a vicious circle that feeds on itself.

Research indicates that there are also several direct ways in which adrenal fatigue can cause depression. High cortisol levels make a person more susceptible to depression and the aftereffects of a traumatic event. Serotonin is a major brain neurotransmitter involved in managing depression, anxiety, and the feeling of well-being. DHEA is involved with managing bad memories and trauma. Addressing adrenal fatigue may be the easiest and most effective way to manage depression, even if it is not the primary cause. A depressed person with more energy and proper hormonal and neurotransmitter balance is more much likely to benefit from therapy or medications. Addressing adrenal fatigue is a great first step for anyone with depression.

Pain

Pain is a major complaint in every physician's office. Most types of pain people experience — such as pain from bruises, rashes, or arthritic changes — are easy to diagnose. The difficult cases are the ones who appear to have pain for no particular reason — no trauma, no lab findings, and no visible indicators. This is when adrenal fatigue needs to be taken into account. When a patient's pain does not have any obvious signs, looking a little deeper into their past history and other health complaints will often reveal adrenal fatigue.

Adrenal fatigue and pain are nearly impossible to separate. Pain is part physical and part emotional, both of which are heavily influenced by the adrenal hormones. I have found that pain is a good indicator of how far the adrenal fatigue has progressed in a person. Cortisol, due to its natural anti-inflammatory qualities, has been shown to be higher in people who minimize their pain levels, which is seen in the early stage of adrenal fatigue. DHEA is a protective hormone that helps the mind to heal after traumatic event. This is also seen in the early stages of adrenal fatigue. A strong indicator that you have reached the end stage of adrenal fatigue is when you can no longer manage your physical pain and subsequently become emotionally overwhelmed. Early-stage adrenal fatigue is marked by higher adrenal hormone levels. Greater hormones levels give you the tools to manage and deal with emotional and physical trauma. The later stages of adrenal fatigue are marked by ever-decreasing hormone levels, making every emotional and physical event feel more dramatic and severe. Pain that has no obvious cause is often the result of the adrenal glands fatiguing and losing the ability to deal with everyday physical aches and pains.

There are several specific biochemical mechanisms that govern how adrenal fatigue leads to pain. In the early stages of adrenal fatigue,high cortisol levels damage collagen fibers, weakening tendons and ligaments. Weak tendons and ligaments lead to weaker muscles, looser joints, and systemic body inflammation. Later stages of adrenal fatigue are marked by lower cortisol levels which reduce the body's ability to fight inflammation. Serotonin is a neurotransmitter produced by the adrenals to control the autonomic nervous system, but it is also used by the brain. Low levels of serotonin in the brain have been linked to depression and increased pain sensitivity.

When pain has no specific cause, adrenal fatigue should always be considered. Adrenal fatigue can be involved in either the physical orthe emotional aspects of the affliction a person is experiencing, and it is likely to be involved in both. One to two percent of all Americans are addicted to prescription pain medications, because the root of their pain is never addressed. Addressing adrenal fatigue is part of the solution.

There are numerous symptoms, conditions, and complaints in which adrenal fatigue is involved. The following section will give a quick overview of how and why.

Perimenopause / Hot Flashes

The end stage of adrenal fatigue causes reduced hormone production in the adrenal glands, which affects perimenopause in two specific ways: 1) indirectly, by reducing the production of DHEA which is used by the ovaries to produce hormones, and 2) directly, by reducing the amount of sexual hormones the adrenal glands produce. Perimenopause symptoms are a key sign that a person has adrenal fatigue. When adrenal fatigue is treated, perimenopause symptoms disappear without the negative side effects of hormone replacement therapy.

Headaches / Migraines

The average American suffers with one headache a month. A more frequent occurrence is an indicator of a health problem. Adrenal fatigue should always be considered in chronic headaches of all types. There are several ways the adrenal glands may be involved in headaches. The adrenal glands are the major regulator of vascular blood flow, which is the cause of pain in most headaches. They may cause collagen weakness, which triggers headaches, and they are involved with moods, which are a leading cause of headaches. I have found that chiropractic care combined with nutritional support for the adrenal glands will eliminate ninety-five percent of even the worst headaches and migraines within eight weeks.

Frequent Urination / Overactive Bladder

When a person finds themself urinating frequently, the adrenals are almost always involved. When a prostate problem or infection is ruled out as a cause of frequent urination, it is time to start a nutritional program to relieve adrenal fatigue. The adrenal hormones are responsible for reabsorbing minerals and water from the kidneys. When adrenal fatigue occurs, the reduced production of hormones leads to increased urination.

Poor Libido in Men and Women

A poor libido is a major complaint I hear in my office from men and women, and proper adrenal gland function is the key to a strong libido. The adrenal glands can affect a person's sexual drive both physically and emotionally. The adrenals produce a hormone group called androgens, which are involved in the production of male and female hormones. DHT is an androgen that has a more powerful effectthan testosterone on men's and women's sexual drives. The adrenal hormones also control vascular blood flow, which is important for an erection and sexual arousal. A strong libido can only take place when a person can manage their stress and anxiety, an area in which the adrenals play an important role.

The Importance of Addressing Adrenal Fatigue

There are so many diseases and symptoms associated with adrenal fatigue that it is impossible to mention them all. It is the vast variety and severity of symptoms that make it both very difficult for physicians to diagnose and very important for them to consider. The important point of this chapter is that if you are not feeling well either emotionally or physically, adrenal fatigue is an issue that needs to be examined as an underlying cause. Every illness is not caused by adrenal fatigue, but every illness is helped by addressing adrenal fatigue. Chronic physical pain and emotional stress are known to cause adrenal fatigue, so ignoring their relevance in the healing process is a recipe for failure.

Dianne

Before going to Dr. Zodkoy, I was miserable. I had so many symptoms that were contributing to me generally feeling "off." I was tired all the time but still had insomnia. I was depressed, achy, and had migraines. Some days, I couldn't go to work, because I didn't have the energy to get out of bed. It felt as if everything was an effort, and an ordinary task would sound overwhelming to me. It reached a point where I had to consider the possibility of going on disability.

Because I had aches in my back, hands, joints, and legs, I went to an orthopedist. He wanted to perform a series of tests, and if each came back negative, he thought it was fibromyalgia.

After being diagnosed with fibromyalgia, I started taking a muscle relaxer. At the same time, I went on Imitrex (sumatriptan) for my migraines and Cymbalta®(duloxetine) for depression. All of these medications had side effects. Mostly, they made me tired. This was a problem, because I was battling tiredness to begin with. There's always the concern of what these medications do to my liver as well.

On a Wednesday, I went to see Dr. Zodkoy, and he diagnosed me with adrenal fatigue syndrome. By Friday, I had no pain. I was sleeping better than I had in years!

A month later, I'm still on the supplements, I'm eating right, and I'm going to the gym. I have no pain at all. Dr. Zodkoy is a miracle worker.

My muscle relaxers are right on my night table beside my bed; I haven't touched them. I'm disappointed that so many people are taking these drugs that are harmful to their bodies, when there are supplements available that work even better! Dr. Zodkoy is so professional and confident in his work. Other people feeling ill don't have to be miserable!

Chapter Five
Adrenal Fatigue Physical Exam and Lab Testing

Obstacles to Proper Diagnosis

Proper diagnosis of adrenal fatigue is based on a patient's history, questionnaire, physical exam, and lab results. A patient's history and questionnaire are the most significant parts to properly diagnosing adrenal fatigue, and their importance is another reason why adrenal fatigue is often misdiagnosed. A thorough patient history takes time, and few physicians want to take the time to do a complete history. Most focus solely on the major area of pain. A patient's physical exam findings are a great way to confirm a diagnosis of adrenal fatigue. Lab testing is also useful and has the advantage of quantifying the problem and providing a method to measure a patient's progress. The most important aspect of diagnosing adrenal fatigue is the patient's story, revealed through their history and questionnaire answers.

One of the biggest problems with getting the proper diagnosis of adrenal fatigue is that standard blood and urine lab tests are not designed to show the problem. Most patients with adrenal fatigue have normal standard lab test results, so their primary physician passes them on to a specialist. A specialist will order more tests, will also find very little wrong, and will either pass the patient on to another physician or misdiagnose the patient. Even if your primary physician was willing to discuss adrenal fatigue, they would not know which tests to order. Remember, adrenal fatigue is not a medical diagnosis but instead a state of dysfunction. America's healthcare system only diagnoses and treats diseases, not dysfunctions.

The newest side of healthcare is called functional medicine. Physicians who practice functional medicine are more concerned with how well the body is functioning and less concerned about naming the disease that causes a symptom. Functional medicine physicians recognize that diseases and symptoms are merely the signs of a poorly functioning body and that the best way to help a patient is to address the dysfunction. Adrenal fatigue is an example of a dysfunction of the body. Functional medicine physicians can be MDs, DCs, DDSs, kinesiologists, or experts in any medical field; it is their awareness and ability to diagnose dysfunction in the body that sets them apart.

The average physician has no understanding of adrenal fatigue, most likely does not accept it as a true diagnosis, and has no idea of how to determine if a patient has it. In an effort to placate patients inquiring about adrenal fatigue, I have seen countless physicians (unfamiliar with adrenal fatigue) mistakenly order a single blood cortisol level test, the results of which are almost always within normal range. The physicians then declare that the patients do not have adrenal fatigue and go back to writing them prescriptions for conditions that they do not have.

Proper diagnosis of adrenal fatigue requires putting together a very specific picture involving your history, questionnaire, physical findings, and specific lab work. If that sounds like a lot of work for your doctor—it is! I believe that many patients are misdiagnosed because physicians do not have the time to properly examine and diagnose a patient in the six to eight minutes allotted by insurance companies.

The final obstacle to diagnosis of adrenal fatigue is related to insurance reimbursement. Since adrenal fatigue is not a recognized diagnosis, the lab testing, medical visits, and treatment are often not paid for by insurance companies. Physicians are often limited to treating only those conditions that are covered under their contract with the insurance company. Physicians can be severely penalized if they venture outside the parameters of their contract by investigating uncommon conditions, referring for non-standard lab tests, or diagnosing a functional health issue like adrenal fatigue.

While the medical and financial obstacles to getting diagnosed properly with adrenal fatigue are numerous, overcoming these obstacles is well worth the effort. Adrenal fatigue is such a major issue in so many patients'conditions that I often start my patients on a nutritional program to improve their adrenal function right after their history and physical exam. Nearly every patient begins to respond to the program even before their lab results return. Every goal worth reaching has a few obstacles in its way, and good health is the ultimate goal.

Questionnaires

A questionnaire is an excellent way to determine if you are suffering from adrenal fatigue. The list of questions in Chapter Oneshould have given you a good indication of whether or not your health issues are stemming from adrenal fatigue. Many patients are convinced that they have adrenal fatigue once they complete the question section of this book. Seeing their main complaint listed along with many of their minor problems is a powerful indicator and motivator.

The questions used in this book are similar to the ones I use when working with the military, in my clinical practice, and when conducting research. These questionnaires are an extremely effective screening tool used by government agencies, the military, and private businesses to monitor workers for burnout in high-stress jobs. Questionnaires have the advantage of being quick, reliable, reproducible, and affordable.

There is a questionnaire called the *Maslach Burnout Inventory* (MBI) (available for a fee at www.MindGarden.com) which has been clinically tested and correlated to problems with the adrenal functions. A study completed at Yale University in cooperation with the United States Navy entitled, *The Impact of Burnout on Human Physiology and on Operational Performance: A Prospective Study of Soldiers Enrolled in the Combat Diver Qualification Course* clearly linked low adrenal function with positive indicators on the questionnaire and multiple health complaints. This particular study clearly showed how a questionnaire can be a good indicator of the results expected on a clinical lab test. Because your questionnaire score is an accurate gauge of how well the adrenals are functioning, it is a valuable tool in monitoring your progress.

The changes you feel over the next few months will correspond to your answers when you retest yourself on the questions in chapter one. Your score decreasing is a good indicator that your adrenals are regaining control and function. There are several physical and lab teststhat can be done by a knowledgeable physician to aid in determining if you have adrenal fatigue. The important and difficult part is finding a knowledgeable physician.

Physical Exam Tests to Diagnose Adrenal Fatigue

A thorough physical exam by a physician familiar with adrenal fatigue is useful in confirming a diagnosis of adrenal fatigue. While a questionnaire can give you the black-and-white score of whether or not you have adrenal fatigue, a physician can examine the nuances. A patient can forget to tell the physician something, make a mistake on a questionnaire, or downplay the severity of their issue, but there is no denying the findings of a physical exam. The other reason physical exam findings are so important is that they can detect the earlier signs of adrenal fatigue, even before multiple symptoms listed on the questionnaire begin to show. The following physical exam findings will help your physician determine if adrenal fatigue is involved in your health complaints.

Pupil Response Test

We have all seen on television when a paramedic looks into an injured person's eyes, shines a light, and notes, "Pupils are fixed and dilated." In medicine, this indicates that the patient is not responsive to the light stimulus and has probably suffered a major injury. That same test can be utilized by a trained physician to determine if your adrenals are functioning normally.

The adrenal glands are responsible for what is known as the pupil response. The pupil response is very simple: When a light is shined in either eye, both pupils will constrict and hold the constriction. If there is no response at all, it can mean severe brain damage, but with adrenal fatigue, there is usually a muted response.

The pupil response test is done in several steps. First, the physician looks at the patient's eyes in a lit room. The pupils should be about forty percent of the iris (the iris is the colorful part of the eye, and the pupil is the dark center). A patient with adrenal fatigue will usually have an enlarged pupil, often taking up to seventy percent of the iris.

The second part of the test involves shining a penlight into one of the eyes in a darkened room and noting the response. The pupils are designed to expand in a dark room, allowing more light to reach the retina, thereby improving a person's night vision. A normal response to having a light shone into the eyes in a dark room is the immediate constriction of the pupil and the holding of the constriction. Adrenal fatigue sufferers will often have an immediate constriction of the pupils, but the physician will quickly begin to see the pupils start to struggle to hold the constriction and then actually begin to expand. This is indicative of adrenal fatigue.

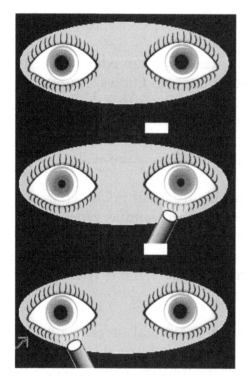

Normal Pupil Size

Normal Pupil Response There is pupil constriction due to a light stimulus.

Abnormal Pupil Response There is no pupil constriction with a light stimulus. This is an indicator of adrenal fatigue.

A more advanced pupil response test can also be performed. A doctor can select any strong muscle in the body to test. The doctor then shines a penlight into the patient's eye and simultaneously retests the muscle in a dim or darkened room. A patient with adrenal fatigue will find that their muscle weakens when they are exposed to a shining penlight. A healthy patient will have no change in muscle strength when stressed by a shining penlight.

Patients who respond poorly to the pupil reflex tests have a very good chance of having adrenal fatigue. They also often complain about the difficulty of driving at night, spots in their vision, dizziness, lightheadedness, and light-induced migraines.

Ligament Laxity Test

The ligament laxity test is simple to perform and demonstrates why so many adrenal fatigue patients have symptoms like joint pain, muscle pains, fibromyalgia, chronic pain syndrome (CPS), and headaches. A physician must first find a strong muscle to test, preferably one that is not involved in the area of pain. The physician then gently tugs on a joint that the muscle crosses and retests the muscles. A patient with adrenal fatigue will find that their muscles will go weak after the tug. A patient without adrenal fatigue will have no change in their muscle strength.

Health Note: If you awaken with a headache, you probably have ligament laxity. The reason is that during the day, your muscles stabilize your neck, but when the muscles relax at night, the ligament laxity allows the joints in the neck to move too much. Excessive movement in the neck leads to pain and also headaches upon awaking. This condition will never heal until the adrenal fatigue is addressed.

The biochemical mechanisms behind the ligament laxity test involve two adrenal pathways. The first part involves the collagen fibers in the ligaments, tendons, and joints of the body. High cortisol levels in the early stages of adrenal fatigue slow down the normal repairs of these parts. Late adrenal fatigue is marked by higher inflammation, which causes additional damage to collagen fibers. The second part involved is the fight-or-flight mechanism, which is momentarily delayed by adrenal fatigue.

The ligament laxity test is an effective way to test for adrenal fatigue, and it demonstrates how adrenal fatigue causes pain and weakness. A person who cannot pass the ligament laxity test will typically have transient pain, arthritis, headaches, fibromyalgia, joint pain, sprains, spasms, and strains. These physical complaints occur because the person's ligaments are not strong enough to stabilize the joints of the body. This ligament instability has the dual effect of causing inflammation in the joints as well as muscle fatigue and strain. Ligament laxity forces muscles to work harder, which leads to strain, spasms, and fibromyalgia. It also makes joints loose, leading to sprains, tendonitis, and bursitis.

Health Note: Patients with chronic neck, shoulder, or low back spasms usually have adrenal fatigue as their hidden diagnosis. Ligaments and tendons are supposed to be the primary joint stabilizers. When patients with adrenal fatigue develop ligament laxity, muscles must then take over the job of joint stability. This constant engagement of the muscle fibers leads to spasms.

If you visit a physician for pain in your muscles or joints, and they do not check for ligament laxity, then you have wasted your time and energy. Unless ligament laxity from adrenal fatigue is ruled out, any diagnosis given to you is only describing your symptoms and is not addressing the underlying cause.

Since the care you will receive for that diagnosis will treat the symptom and not the cause, you may receive some temporary relief from that symptom, but your overall health will not be better, and another symptom will shortly arrive. It takes only a few minutes for a physician to check for ligament laxity, but the answers can affect your entire life.

Orthostatic Hypotension

Orthostatic hypotension is also known as postural hypotension, orthostasis, and colloquially as a head rush or dizzy spell. It describes the transient low blood pressure that occurs in some people when they change positions. The change in position is usually from a low-gravity position, like lying down or reclining, to a higher gravity position, like standing. Medically, it is defined as a fall in systolic blood pressure of at least 20 mmHg and diastolic blood pressure of at least 10 mmHg when a person assumes a standing position. This temporary but significant drop in blood pressure reduces the blood flow to the brain and can cause the symptoms of dizziness, vertigo, blacking out, or fainting.

The test for orthostatic hypotension is very simple. The blood pressure of a patient is taken in the lying down position and then in the standing position. There should be no significant difference in the two readings, (a significant change being a drop of 10 or more points). I also find it important to notice how the patient rises from the table. A patient who moves slowly to avoid dizziness and one who rises quickly and wobbles are both offering a great clue to their condition. This exemplifies the fact that it is not just the test results that are of value in diagnosing a condition.

Physicians will often diagnose this condition as low blood pressure, minor dehydration, old age, or a secondary reaction to a medication. It amazes me how few physicians check a patient for orthostatic hypotension even when a patient describes the problem to them. None of the above conditions or any of the other misdiagnoses physicians give out for this condition are the same as orthostatic hypotension. It is a dysfunction of the body's ability to maintain normal pressure when gravity is taken into account, and none of the other conditions are affected the same way.

Health Hint: If you find that you are dizzy when you rise from a lying or sitting position, you probably have orthostatic hypotension caused by adrenal fatigue.

The reason adrenal fatigue causes orthostatic hypotension is that your blood vessels must contract quickly and forcefully to keep your blood pressure stable. Adrenal fatigue reduces the blood vessels' contractile strength and response. The symptoms of dizziness, headaches, dimmed vision, vertigo, and fainting all occur from the loss of blood going to the brain.

Generalized Stress Response Test

The generalized stress response test varies by physician and by a patient's complaints. The objective of this test is to determine how the patient's adrenal glands react to a stressor that is unique to that person. These tests all rely on the doctor testing a strong muscle and then evoking a stressor to see if the muscle changes strength. Patients with adrenal fatigue will become weak when a stressful event occurs. This testing procedure is excellent for determining specific stressors to a patient which will be important in developing a desensitization program for them in the future.

Several Examples of General Stress Response Testing:
A patient who has symptoms of adrenal fatigue and complains

of sensitivity to loud noises may be tested by being exposed to loud noises.

A patient who has symptoms of adrenal fatigue and complains they feel worse after a stressful event, like driving, may be tested by being startled by a sudden clap or tap.

A patient who has symptoms of adrenal fatigue and complains of difficulty going to sleep may be tested lying down in the dark.

A patient who has symptoms of adrenal fatigue and complains of joint pain after exercise may be tested by doing a few minutes of exercise.

Testing a patient's specific area of complaint for adrenal fatigue involvement is an excellent way to pick up early cases of adrenal fatigue. It also helps a patient understand how their specific problem is directly related to adrenal fatigue.

Full Inspiration Test

Through the years, I have found that the most common physical sign of early adrenal fatigue is pain in the neck and mid back, directly under the shoulder blade. Many patients had been treated by numerous orthopedists, physical therapists, and chiropractors for this problem but received only minor relief. The reason this problem does not respond to care is because it is often misdiagnosed as a muscle spasm, but it is actually a strain of the rib joint. The rib joint is the spot where the ribs attach to the spine, and it tends to be the most vulnerable joint to adrenal fatigue.

The full inspiration test is based on a finding that people with adrenal fatigue tend to have weakness in the joint that attaches the ribs to the spine. The test is done in two parts. First, the patient takes a very deep breath. If this causes the patient pain, it is a good indication of a rib strain. Second, a physician tests a strong muscle and then retests the muscle with the patient holding a deep breath. A positive test is indicated by a previously strong muscle being weakened during full inspiration. The full inspiration test is not specific to adrenal fatigue, but it is another clue to proper diagnosis.

The physical exam tests for adrenal fatigue are all based on stimulating the body so that the adrenal glands are pushed to respond. It is the adrenal glands' inability to respond to the stressors that indicates there is an issue that needs to be addressed. A single positive finding is not enough to diagnose adrenal fatigue, but I have found that patients with adrenal fatigue will fail at least a few of the physical tests that are administered.

The physical exam tests listed above, in conjunction with your history and questionnaire, are often enough information to properly diagnose adrenal fatigue. In my clinic, if enough of the above signs are positive, I will begin treatment before I get the lab test results back. Adrenal fatigue responds so quickly to proper care that often the patient will feel dramatic results before the test results (which typically take ten days) are returned. Lab results are useful for specific cases, but not necessary for all cases.

Lab Testing for Adrenal Fatigue

The remainder of this chapter will go through some clinical lab tests that can help a physician diagnose adrenal fatigue. While adrenal fatigue can be diagnosed with high accuracy through a simple questionnaire supported by physical exam findings, clinical lab testing is of great value. Clinical lab testing has the advantage of quantifying the degree of the adrenal fatigue and helps in fine tuning the treatment plan. When reading this chapter, just familiarize yourself with the tests and what they indicate. It is not your job to know every detail about the tests; that is the job of your physician.

Lab testing for adrenal fatigue is rarely available at your local clinic or lab. Either you or your physician will need to get a testing kit from a specialty lab and perform the test at home. The tests are both convenient and easy to perform. I use test kits from NeuroScience, Inc., which are affordable and reliable. All of the graphs in this chapter are from NeuroScience test kits.

Health Note:Lab testing is a great tool to use when a patient cannot be seen by a physician.I recently completed a program with the USMC on burnout/resiliency/PTSD and their relationship to adrenal fatigue.Due to the fact that the participants were hundreds or thousands of miles away, lab testing and questionnaires were the only available tools for determining nutritional protocols to improve the health of these Marines. I am proud to say that the average Marine had a reductionin their complaints of over 40 percent in just ninety days.This was accomplished without changing their environment or lifestyle.If a program based on this information can restore combat Marines with life-or-death stressors, I am sure it can work for you.

There are several lab tests that, when ordered by a knowledgeable physician, will indicate adrenal fatigue. While these tests are covered by most insurance companies, they are not typically ordered, so you need a physician who is familiar with the test protocols and interpreting the results. Test results for adrenal fatigue are not as black-and-white as a traditional lab test. Results will determine the amount of hormones the adrenals are producing, and if they are generating the correct amount at the right time. In order to be of use in diagnosing adrenal fatigue, lab testing for the adrenal glands'function must account for the fluctuation in their production throughout the day. Another factor to consider when ordering lab tests for the adrenal glands is which hormones to test, because the adrenal glands produce numerous hormones, and testing all of them is impractical. These complexities in ordering and evaluating lab tests for adrenal fatigue are the reason why most physicians shy away from this diagnosis and instead tend toward an easier misdiagnosis.

Saliva Cortisol Test

Cortisol, a major hormone produced by the adrenal glands, is usually used as the primary indicator hormone for adrenal gland production. The saliva cortisol test measures the amount of cortisol your body is producing. This test requires four saliva samples to be taken throughout the day in order to give an accurate indication of how the adrenal glands are functioning. The reason you need to take four samples is because your cortisol levels should differ by 400 percent from morning to evening. Your cortisol levels (and thus your adrenal production) are highest in the morning, when you need to be energized and ready for life's activities. Adrenal production tapers off dramatically as the day progresses, so that you feel tired, relaxed, and ready to get a good night's rest. When a physician reads your saliva cortisol levels, they are not just looking at *how much* cortisol is produced but *when* it is produced and how much is produced in relationship to the rest of the day. Unless cortisol levels follow a very specific pattern, symptoms will occur.

Figure 1 is a graph of a normal cortisol level test. Cortisol levels are represented by the thick line, and the acceptable ranges are represented by the two thin lines. Cortisol is high in the morning and has a steady decline until late in the evening. This person would awaken refreshed and energized and would be serene when bedtime came around.

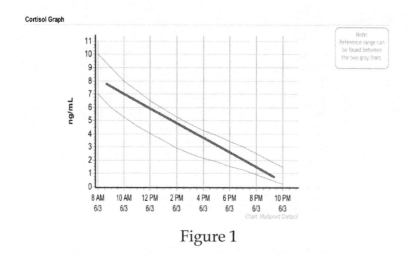

Figure 1

Overproducing Adrenal Glands: The Go-Go-Go Guy

Figure 2 is a common abnormal saliva cortisol level test that I like to call the "go-go-go" guy. A person with this test result is generating a large amount of cortisol all day long. Notice that the thick line that represents cortisol levels is above the reference range. This person thinks they are thriving under stress, but in reality, they are burning out their adrenals and are heading toward a crash. This person is already starting to notice that they don't feel right unless they are being pushed and is probably starting to have difficulty sleeping. This is typical of a person in the early stage of adrenal fatigue, when the adrenals are overproducing hormones to meet the stress the mind and body are under.

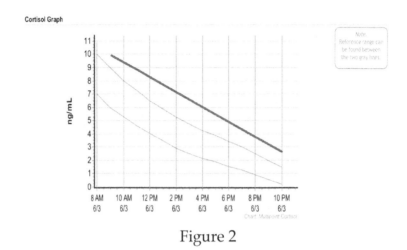

Figure 2

Underproducing Adrenal Glands: Fatigued Out

Figure 3 is an abnormal saliva cortisol level test that I call "fatigued out." This person has little to no change in their cortisol levels, so they feel fatigued all the time, have multiple physical and emotional symptoms, and despite their fatigue, are unable to sleep well. They usually need lots of coffee to get going and have lost their lust for life. Their cortisol levels hit the normal range toward the end of the day, so they usually feel better later in the day. This person usually has depression, anxiety, and pain.

I commonly see this graph in patients suffering from fibromyalgia, PTSD, and end-stage adrenal fatigue, as well as those patients diagnosed with burnout or claiming to be burned out. They blame a lot of their condition on work because of the stress they feel during work hours, which is actually due to a combination of their work stress and their lower daytime cortisol levels.

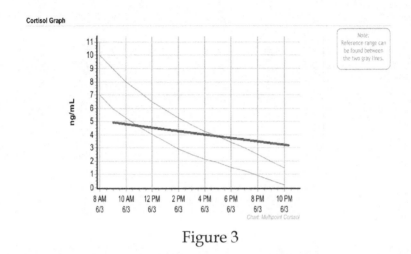

Figure 3

Minimal Cortisol Production: The I'm Done Person

Figure 4 is another common abnormal saliva cortisol level test which represents full adrenal fatigue. This person's cortisol levels are all below normal. They have zero energy, zero drive, depression, pain, confusion, dizziness, and every other symptom under the sun. The "I'm done"person has given up and can barely handle any of life's positive or negative experiences. You can pick any emotional or physical diagnosis, and they will have it.

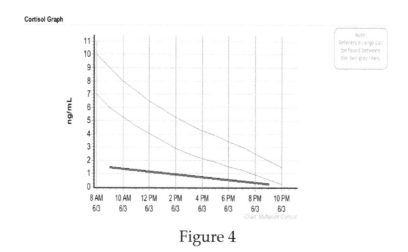

Figure 4

Abnormal Cortisol Pattern: The Night Owl

Figure 5 represents the "night owl" person who has a tough time all day long but perks up at the end of the day. They describe themself as a night owl, because they feel most energized and productive at night. This is commonly seen at the middle stage of adrenal fatigue.

This is probably the most common abnormal saliva cortisol level test. This person has low cortisol levels all day but then swings high at night. This patient is fatigued and listless all day but then cannot fall asleep. Depression and anxiety are almost always seen in these patients.

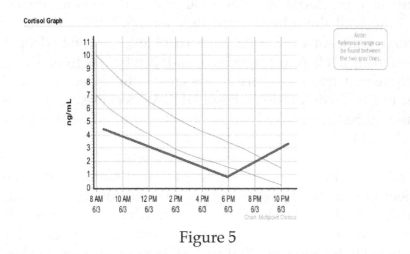

Figure 5

Abnormal cortisol graphs can vary in hundreds of different ways. There can be spikes and dips in the morning, afternoon, or evening. Any change in the normal saliva cortisol levels will cause both physical and emotional symptoms. As you can see, if a physician took only one cortisol level sample, they would miss the abnormal trend in many of the above cases. It is critical that both the level and the trend of your saliva cortisol be considered when being diagnosed.

Saliva DHEA test

Saliva DHEA should be tested at the same time that saliva cortisol level is tested. While it is generally sufficient to have your saliva DHEA tested only one time during the day, usually along with the first cortisol level test of the day, recent research has shown that for difficult cases there is value in measuring saliva DHEA along with saliva cortisol levels at all four intervals. I find that multiple DHEA levels are especially useful for those suffering from any type of PTSD.

The importance of DHEA is twofold: 1) Since DHEA, like cortisol, is produced by the adrenal glands, it gives an indication of how well the adrenals are functioning. DHEA levels will drop significantly lower before cortisol levels begin to drop. By measuring DHEA, a physician can tell what stage of adrenal fatigue you are in. 2) There also is great value in calculating the cortisol to DHEA ratio (cortisol:DHEA), because an abnormal variance has been linked to a greater susceptibility to depression and PTSD.

Cortisol:DHEA has been getting a lot of attention in the latest scientific research. It is becoming a key indicator in documenting PTSD. Cortisol:DHEA also has significance in determining how severe the adrenal fatigue has become. An extremely high cortisol:DHEA indicates that adrenal fatigue is severe and long-standing.

By testing DHEA in conjunction with cortisol, a physician is able to determine if the adrenals are sacrificing production of some hormones in favor of more critical hormones. A high cortisol:DHEA ratio indicates that the body is in a state of chronic stress and is focusing on hormones like cortisol that are involved in dealing with that stress, rather than hormones like DHEA that allow the body to heal from a stressful event. A patient may have fairly normal cortisol levels but low DHEA levels. This would be an early indication of adrenal fatigue and is commonly seen in patients complaining of a low libido, sexual dysfunction, perimenopause, and symptoms of low testosterone.

Health Hint: When you consider how many American women are on female replacement hormones and how many men are on testosterone and erectile dysfunction medications, it is clear how important it is to test DHEA. DHEA nutritional supplementation usually alleviates the symptoms associated with these conditions without side effects. Plus, it is a huge boost to a person's sex drive.

Urine Neurotransmitter Testing

Functional medicine physicians have been treating adrenal fatigue for decades. I myself learned about it over twenty years ago. For past few decades, the focus of testing and treating adrenal fatigue has all been on the adrenal glands themselves. It has only been in the last several years that functional medicine physicians have adopted neurotransmitter testing for the diagnosis and treatment of adrenal fatigue. Neurotransmitter testing allows the physician to see how adrenal fatigue is affecting the nervous system and to better tailor a treatment program.

About Neurotransmitters: Neurotransmitters are chemical compounds released by nerve endings to either stimulate or suppress the nervous system. They are found in the body and the brain. An imbalance in their concentration (either high or low) can cause both physical and emotional symptoms, including anxiety, depression, fibromyalgia, and insomnia. Most anxiety and depression medications work by affecting neurotransmitters in the brain.

Testing for neurotransmitters in the urine can be useful in diagnosing adrenal fatigue. The production of several neurotransmitters — including norepinephrine, epinephrine, and serotonin — begins in the adrenals. Neurotransmitter testing has the added benefit of giving insight into how best to treat the symptoms that accompany adrenal fatigue, like depression, anxiety, fatigue, nervousness, and obsessive-compulsive disorder (OCD). Neurotransmitters are the chemicals that nerves use to talk to each other in the brain and in the body. How you feel, both physically and emotionally, depends on the balance between the stimulation and suppression of the nervous system by neurotransmitters. Most anxiety and depression medications, including SSRIs and monoamine oxidase inhibitors (MAOIs) work on these same neurotransmitters.

Neurotransmitters can be either stimulating or suppressing in nature. In order for a person to be able to manage and respond to emotional and physical stress, there needs to be a balance between the two groups. The same neurotransmitters work in the central nervous system (the brain and spinal column) as well as in the peripheral nervous system (the body, arms, legs, and organs). This is one reason why patients with psychological issues often have physical complaints and vice versa. Neurotransmitters are a key component of the mind-body relationship.

Neurotransmitter and Adrenal Hormone Clinical Correlations

SUPRESSING

Serotonin — plays important roles in mood, sleep, and appetite
High levels:SSRI medications, stress, platelet aggregation
Low levels:low mood, sleep difficulties, uncontrolled appetite, headaches, hot flashes

5-Hydroxyindoleacetic   Acid   (5-HIAA) — the   primary metabolite of serotonin involving monoamine oxidase A (MAO-A) and aldehyde dehydrogenase
High levels:intestinal complaints, upregulated MAO activity
Low levels: no associated clinical symptoms to date

Gamma-Aminobutyric   Acid   (GABA) — primary   inhibitory neurotransmitter in the brain, necessary to feel calm and relaxed
High levels:excessive energy, anxiousness, sleep difficulties, headaches
Low   levels:uncontrolled   excessive   energy,   uncontrolled anxiousness, uncontrolled sleep difficulties, poor impulse control

Taurine — important for proper heart function, healthy sleep, and promoting calmness
High Levels: anxiousness, sleep difficulties, supplementation (example: energy drinks)
Low levels: uncontrolled excessive energy, uncontrolled anxiousness, uncontrolled sleep difficulties, poor impulse control

Glycine — like GABA, helps calm and relax the body
High levels: anxiousness, low mood, stress-related symptoms, high immune activity
Low levels: mood disorders

STIMULATING

Glutamate — primary excitatory neurotransmitter, necessary for learning and memory
High levels: anxiousness, low mood, activated immune system
Low levels: fatigue, learning difficulties

Histamine — helps control sleep-wake cycle, plus energy and motivation
High levels:hypersensitivities, sleep difficulties
Low levels: fatigue, sleep difficulties

Phenethylamine (PEA) — important for focus and concentration
High levels: mind racing, sleep difficulties, anxiousness
Low levels: difficulty paying attention, difficulty thinking clearly, low mood, fatigue

3,4-Dihydroxyphenylacetic Acid (DOPAC) — primary metabolite of dopamine involving monoamine oxidase B (MAO-B) and aldehyde dehydrogenase
High levels: excessive energy, focus issues, developmental delays, upregulated MAO activity, stress
Low levels: no associated clinical symptoms to date

Dopamine—responsible for feelings of pleasure and satisfaction, also muscle control, muscle function, and GI issues
High levels: poor intestinal function, developmental delay, attention issues
Low levels: urges, impulsivity, cravings, movement disorders

Norepinephrine (aka noradrenaline)—important for mental focus, emotional stability, and endocrine function
High levels: anxiousness, stress, excessive energy, high blood pressure
Low Levels: fatigue, lack of focus, lack of motivation, low mood, sleep difficulties, hot flashes, headaches

Epinephrine (aka adrenaline)—important for motivation, energy, and mental focus
High levels: anxiousness, sleep difficulties, attention issues
Low levels: fatigue, low mood, lack of motivation

HORMONES:

Cortisol—primary glucocorticoid, produced by the adrenal gland, regulates body's stress response
High levels: anxiousness, sleep difficulties, low immune activity
Low levels: fatigue, anxiousness

Dehydroepiandrosterone (DHEA)—produced by the adrenal gland,precursor to estrogens and androgens
High levels: anxiousness
Low levels: fatigue, menopause symptoms, low sex hormone levels

Creatinine—a normalizing parameter used to calculate neurotransmitter levels

The preceding is a list of frequently tested neurotransmitters and the effects that either high or low levels have on the mind and body. It should be noted that often too much or too little of any neurotransmitter will cause both physical and emotional symptoms. Because many systems in the body only react in one way, it is common for too much or too little of the same neurotransmitter to cause the same complaints.

Think of your nervous system as a light bulb. With too much light, you are blinded. With too little light, it is dark. But in both cases, you cannot see. The light bulb example explains how neurotransmitters work in the mind and body. You need just the right amount to get proper function without symptoms.

Testing a person's neurotransmitters is useful for anyone with anxiety, depression, or an undiagnosed condition. It is a way to evaluate the function of the nervous system, check the communication between the mind-body link, and get an indication of how best to correct the problem.

The following image displays the results of a neurotransmitter test.

Neurotransmitters produced by the adrenal glands

| Suppressing | Stimulating |

Neurotransmitters

	2.5%	20%	80%	97.5%	Result	Collected	Inter-Quintile Range	Reference Range	Units
Serotonin					179.5	06/03/2012 (9:00AM)	99 - 203	57 - 306	µg/gCr
5-HIAA					4,359.6	06/03/2012 (9:00AM)	1,800 - 5,900	800 - 13000	µg/gCr
GABA					8.8 (H)	06/03/2012 (9:00AM)	3.9 - 7.9	2.4 - 12.7	µMol/gCr
Taurine					187.4	06/03/2012 (9:00AM)	156 - 535	52 - 1025	µMol/gCr
Glycine					2,369.1 (H)	06/03/2012 (9:00AM)	441 - 1258	182 - 2225	µMol/gCr
Glutamate					50.2 (H)	06/03/2012 (9:00AM)	13.5 - 36.8	6.9 - 71.8	µMol/gCr
Histamine					102.2 (H)	06/03/2012 (9:00AM)	10 - 32	4 - 71	µg/gCr
PEA					103.8 (H)	06/03/2012 (9:00AM)	29 - 83	15 - 167	nMol/gCr
Dopamine					525.8 (H)	06/03/2012 (9:00AM)	106 - 191	64 - 261	µg/gCr
DOPAC					1,665.3 (H)	06/03/2012 (9:00AM)	300 - 1000	100 - 2100	µg/gCr
Norepinephrine					133.6 (H)	06/03/2012 (9:00AM)	28 - 51	19 - 76	µg/gCr
Epinephrine					23.3 (H)	06/03/2012 (9:00AM)	7.1 - 13.6	4.7 - 20.8	µg/gCr

Red or light red bars indicate results out of Inter-Quintile Range

Inter-Quintile Range is defined as the 60th percentile.
Reference Range as the 95th percentile

This test indicates that the neurotransmitters involved in stimulating the nervous system (shown below the dividing line) are overactive. The suppressing neurotransmitters (shown above the dividing line) are mostly normal. This person could present as agitated, confused, irritated or anxious, but is most likely to have a combination of these complaints.

The goal of this person's treatment would be to use nutritional supplements to reduce the overstimulation, while preserving the normal suppression levels. Proper nutritional support for this patient will help reduce their emotional and physical complaints without causing any of the typical side effects found with the use of medication.

Retesting of the patient in ninety days will often show that their neurotransmitters have been balanced and their major physical and emotional complaints have been reduced. Treating neurotransmitter imbalances often goes hand in hand with treating adrenal fatigue.

Neurotransmitters correspond extremely well with how a patient is feeling. The following is a before-and-after account of a thirteen-year-old patient who was suffering with an acute onset of severe OCD, anxiety, and mysophobia (a phobia of germs). The patient's condition was so severe that they would sleep in the shower with the water running and walk only on paper towels to avoid germs. After traditional therapy and medications proved ineffective, the patient was referred to my office.

Neurotransmitters

	2.5%	10%	80%	97.5%	Result	Collected	Inter-Quintile Range	Reference Range	Units
Serotonin					**128.8** 265.4 (H)	04/20/2013 (10:00AM) 05/09/2012 (7:00AM)	99 - 203	57 - 306	µg/gCr
5-HIAA					**2,390.4** 2,325.6	04/20/2013 (10:00AM) 05/09/2012 (7:00AM)	1800 - 5900	800 - 13000	µg/gCr
GABA					**5.8** 9.1 (H)	04/20/2013 (10:00AM) 05/09/2012 (7:00AM)	3.9 - 7.9	2.4 - 12.7	µmol/gCr
Taurine					**305.0** 254.2	04/20/2013 (10:00AM) 05/09/2012 (7:00AM)	156 - 535	52 - 1025	µmol/gCr
Glycine					**1,077.8** 439.5 (L)	04/20/2013 (10:00AM) 05/09/2012 (7:00AM)	441 - 1258	182 - 2225	µmol/gCr
Glutamate					**33.0** 32.9	04/20/2013 (10:00AM) 05/09/2012 (7:00AM)	13.5 - 36.8	6.9 - 71.8	µmol/gCr
Histamine					**13.4** 35.1 (H)	04/20/2013 (10:00AM) 05/09/2012 (7:00AM)	10 - 32	4 - 71	µg/gCr
PEA					**32.2** 68.0	04/20/2013 (10:00AM) 05/09/2012 (7:00AM)	29 - 83	15 - 167	nmol/gCr
Dopamine					**174.8** 243.4 (H)	04/20/2013 (10:00AM) 05/09/2012 (7:00AM)	106 - 191	64 - 261	µg/gCr
DOPAC					**815.5**	04/20/2013 (10:00AM)	575 - 1140	360 - 1800	µg/gCr
Norepinephrine					**35.1** 63.6 (H)	04/20/2013 (10:00AM) 05/09/2012 (7:00AM)	28 - 51	19 - 76	µg/gCr
Epinephrine					**6.6 (L)** 11.2	04/20/2013 (10:00AM) 05/09/2012 (7:00AM)	7.1 - 13.6	4.7 - 20.8	µg/gCr

Red or light red bars indicate results out of Inter-Quintile Range.
Previous results are printed below current results in a lighter red or gray.
Range change effective 4/1/2013 for the following parameters: DOPAC

594563

Inter-Quintile Range is defined as the 60th percentile.
Reference Range as the 95th percentile.

The test results shown here list the neurotransmitters with two bars to the right of each one. The bottom bar is the original test, and the top bar is the retest. The patient's original test showed that half of the neurotransmitters were out of balance. The nervous system was overloaded and sending too many signals. This overload had led to the patient's bizarre behavior.

These results are typical of someone who is being overstimulated. The patient's stimulating neurotransmitters — dopamine, histamine, and norepinephrine — were causing too much stimulation. The body's response was to overproduce the suppressing neurotransmitters, GABA and serotonin. The result was the acute development of psychological symptoms.

Proper treatment involved supporting the adrenals so that they could: 1) handle the stress that had triggered the stimulating neurotransmitters, 2) downregulate the stimulating neurotransmitters, and 3) aid in the production of suppressing neurotransmitters.

The results were amazing. Within days, the patient began to return to normal and was nearly back to their old ways in less than a month. The follow-up neurotransmitter tests showed that the patient's return to normalcy was mirrored by the return of their neurotransmitters to regular levels.

This case is an excellent example of how a patient's symptoms may only be indicated on a neurotransmitter test, which makes it ideal for patients who know there is something wrong but yet they keep getting misdiagnosed.

When neurotransmitters are tested on adrenal fatigue sufferers, there are several patterns that show up. These patterns serve as good indicators of what stage of adrenal fatigue a person is in and how best to treat them. Two of the most common patterns are the "fidgeter" and the "downer."

The Fidgeter

This person typically appears as overactive, fidgety, and nervous. They are overexcited, overstimulated, and have high levels of nearly all of their neurotransmitters. They often feel overwhelmed at home, school, and work, despite the fact that the actual stress level is minimal. This is very common in attention deficit disorder (ADD), attention deficit hyperactivity disorder (ADHD), psychosomatics, and those with addictive tendencies. This person is typically in the middle stages of adrenal fatigue, when the adrenal glands are still able to overproduce hormones, but symptoms are starting to occur. This person is often overstimulated more through their own nervous system and thoughts than from external stressors.

The Downer

This person is chronically down or depressed. They don't even get excited when things are good. They tend to be sad, fatigued, and disengaged. They will often comment that they have little interest in friends, activities, or life in general. This person's neurotransmitter levels are usually all very low, as are their adrenal levels. This type of person is in the end stage of adrenal fatigue.

Finding a Physician

The greatest difficulty in testing for adrenal fatigue is finding a physician who is qualified and knowledgeable enough about how to perform these tests and properly interpret their results. The failure of the medical profession to accept that the adrenal glands can become fatigued is what has prohibited most medical physicians from even exploring the tests to determine the status of the adrenal glands. There are chiropractors, acupuncturists, and alternative medical physicians who can do these tests, and with a little work, you can find someone near you. I have included a reference section at the back of this book to aid your search.

Joe

For a long time, I was feeling the worst I had ever felt in my whole life. I was tired all the time, felt run down, weakened, and had struggled with terrible digestive issues for two years. The condition was so limiting that I had no desire to do anything or engage in any activities. It was also affecting my demeanor. I was often moody, because I was just so tired. Everyday tasks were a struggle for me, so I allowed for things to fall by the wayside, while I lived a very sedentary lifestyle. I was miserable.

My stomach issues were very debilitating, so I went to a couple of gastroenterologists at Robert Wood Johnson University Hospital. These doctors ran a battery of tests, including a colonoscopy, endoscopy, and blood work to test for celiac disease and bacteria. Nothing came up positive.

It was at that point that my psychologist, whom I was seeing for stress issues, recommended Dr. Zodkoy. I explained to Dr. Zodkoy that I had just gone through a divorce and had other stressors in my life. He explained that this amount of intense stress can lead to an illness known as adrenal burnout.

Dr. Zodkoy took the time to explain that the more stress a person has, the more the glands get taxed and have to overproduce. Then, they underproduce and leave the person feeling run-down and tired. He put me on supplements to support the adrenal glands and health. These supplements would also make sure that my hormones are all producing correctly.

I have been seeing Dr. Zodkoy for several weeks now and am feeling 75 percent better. I went from not being able to do the dishes to signing up for martial arts classes — something I couldn't even dream of three weeks ago. After exhausting all traditional medicines, I went to Dr. Zodkoy with an open mind, and now I'm so glad that I did.

Chapter Six
Healing Adrenal Fatigue

A Comprehensive Treatment Program

By now, I hope I've made it clear to you that adrenal fatigue is a complex problem with multiple causes and symptoms involving your mind, body, and environment. The difficulties in treating adrenal fatigue are compounded by the following factors: it is often impossible to completely separate yourself from the stressors; there is no magical drug cure; and it is poorly understood by your physician and family. The good news is that adrenal fatigue, once properly diagnosed, begins to respond to proper treatment in just a few weeks. The program that I have created will help you to resolve your symptoms and restore your overall physical and emotional health. Treatment for your adrenal fatigue is the first step in improving your entire life.

Over the last twenty years in practice, I have treated thousands of patients with adrenal fatigue. I have a lot of experience treating patients in my office and from thousands of miles away. The program I created takes all of that experience into account. Here are several key points to keep in mind when starting on a treatment plan for adrenal fatigue:

- Doing something is better than doing nothing. This plan has been concentrated to include the most critical points, sacrificing an ideal program for a doable program.

- It takes time to adjust to the program, so give yourself

several weeks to experience a change.

- Don't stop because you feel better. Once the adrenal glands have been fatigued, you need to maintain your lifestyle changes and nutritional support, or your symptoms will slowly return.

- If all other serious conditions have been ruled out by a physician,it is safe to start the program without being tested.

- Using a scale of 1-10, keep a chart of your physical and emotional complaints. Rate yourself daily or several times a week to monitor your progress.

Adrenal fatigue affects the physical, mental, and chemical aspects of the body. To properly heal and not just alleviate symptoms, a treatment program will need to address all three factors. Each step of my protocol is designed to benefit the mental, physical, and chemical interactions of the body. For example, changing your diet to be more alkaline will reduce the inflammation in your joints (chemical); improve your muscle tone and reduce your weight (physical); and increase your Vitamin B intake, which improves mental focus and outlook (mental). This program is designed so that every step you take to improve your adrenal fatigue will also improve your overall health.

Many of my adrenal fatigue patients tell me that they have tried chiropractic, physical therapy, acupuncture, psychotherapy, nutritionists, yoga, and more, with either temporary relief or no relief. The reason that these treatments failed is because none of them by themselves are strong enough to heal the physical, emotional, and biochemical damage caused by adrenal fatigue. When treating adrenal fatigue, you need to use a variety of treatment methods simultaneously to insure you are healing all aspects of the problem. A single treatment method is designed to address a specific symptom. The synergy of the physical, emotional, and biochemical careis what allows for full and complete healing.

I have been treating patients for over twenty years, and I realize that your only concern right now is getting rid of your symptoms. The idea of overhauling your life doesn't seem possible, but let's go through the steps anyway. If you can commit a few weeks to starting the program, I am sure that your body will start to heal, and your symptoms will begin to lessen. While it can take up to a year to fully recover, adrenal fatigue sufferers usually begin to feel a change in just a week or two. When you imagine yourself as a healthier and happier person, living a much longer and more productive life, the end results are worth the journey.

Health Note: Visualization is an excellent way to help your mind focus on the healing process. Take a few quiet minutes in the morning to focus on how you want to feel. This simple process will remind you of why you are on this program and help guide your mind and body to your ultimate goal of good health.

The single most important goal of treating adrenal fatigue is restoring your body back to homeostasis, or balance. You cannot completely eliminate the stressors from your life, but you can make your body better able to handle and adapt to them. A body that can adapt to acute and chronic stressors will not develop adrenal fatigue nor suffer from the accompanying emotional and physical symptoms. Strengthening the body so that it maintains normal function while under stress, rather than either over or undercompensating, is the key to long-term, optimum health.

Nutritional Support for Adrenal Fatigue

I am starting with the nutritional aspect of the adrenal fatigue healing program, because it offers the fastest, easiest, and most effective results. The nutritional approach to healing adrenal fatigue involves dietary changes and nutritional supplements. I have never found a patient to recover from adrenal fatigue without nutritional supplements. Dietary changes are also important, but I have seen adrenal fatigue sufferers who have excellent diets and still have adrenal issues. While I often use sophisticated lab testing in my office to determine the exact nutritional support a patient requires, I have found that adrenal fatigue sufferers almost always need the same baseline nutritional supplements to start. Beginning a program with these simple and safe supplements often offers dramatic and rapid relief.

It is easy to become overwhelmed with all the different nutritional supplements that can be used for adrenal fatigue, but don't worry—just relax—it is really very easy. When deciding on which nutritional supplements to use for adrenal fatigue, think more general than specific. Many nutritional supplements are synergistic in nature, and when taken together, a lower dosage may achieve the same or greater effect. You do not have to pick the "right"one, just one that allows the body to heal itself. The reason I have been successful in treating the most difficult cases is not because of my genius but because of the body's genius. If you give the body nutritionally rich foods and nutritional supplements that focus on the dysfunctional area, the body can and will heal itself. One of the best ways to ensure that you are using the right nutritional supplement is to use a product that has a combination of synergistic ingredients.

Note that I have not included recommended dosages for the suggested nutritional supplements. Without knowing the specifics of the product, such as how it was made, the quality of the raw material, the ingredients, and whether it is a capsule or tablet, it is impossible to give a dosage range for nutritional supplements. I have instead chosen to include (in the resource chapter in the back of the book) specific nutritional supplements. These nutritional supplements are many of the same products I have used in my office for years with great success and safety. The dosages recommend on these products have been beneficial to my patients for decades.

Adrenal fatigue can be treated to such a great extent that many sufferers believe the issue has been corrected. I have found that adrenal fatigue is rarely cured but more often put into remission. It is important that once you start to feel better, you keep with your new lifestyle habits and maintain nutritional supplementation to avoid a relapse. Your new lifestyle and nutritional supplements will not only help you fight off adrenal fatigue but also other diseases of aging, like cardiac disease, arthritis, and poor memory.

Adaptogens

Adaptogens are nutritional supplements, usually herbal-based, which have been shown to help the body adapt to changes in physical, emotional, and biochemical stress. While the concept of using adaptogens or herbal remedies is unusual in the United States, it is common practice throughout Europe, Asia, and the rest of the world. Adaptogens have been studied and shown to help with a variety of emotional, physical, and biochemical stressors, which makes them ideal for healing a complex issue like adrenal fatigue. Much of the original work on adaptogens was done in the former Soviet Union in the 1960's through the 1990's and was believed to be a major factor in their sports dominance during that era.

Health Note of Interest: Americans tend to think that we have the latest and greatest health care. The truth is that much of the world is ahead of the United States when it comes to healthcare involving disease prevention and quality of life. While the United States spends more money and a greater percentage of our gross domestic budget on health care, we get very poor returns. The World Health Organization regularly ranks the United States below thirty other countries in quality of life, infant mortality, and life expectancy — often behind developing and underdeveloped countries. Other countries often adapt innovative and cost-effective methods to improve and maintain their citizens' health. For example, Russia has been providing radial keratotomy eye surgery (the basis of laser eye surgery) since 1974 — a full decade before it was common in the United States! Another example is that Scandinavian countries offer their citizens massages as part of their health system.

Adaptogens may not be common in American medicine, but they are recognized by the U.S. Food and Drug Administration (FDA). The FDA has recognized adaptogens as a functional term in medicine since 1998. A nutritional supplement needs to meet certain criteria to be considered an adaptogen.

According to the original definition of an adaptogen:

- the adaptogenic effect is nonspecific in that the adaptogen increases resistance to a very broad spectrum of harmful factors ("stressors") of different physical, chemical, and biological natures;

- an adaptogen is to have a normalizing effect, that is, it counteracts or prevents disturbances brought about by stressors; and

- an adaptogen must be innocuous and have a broad range of therapeutic effects without causing any disturbance (other than very marginal) to the normal functioning of the organism.

Doesn't the above definition of an adaptogen read just like what you need to restore your overall health?

Adaptogens are a new class of nutritional supplements that have been shown to restore the homeostasis of the body in response to emotional, physical, and biochemical stressors without doing any harm. Adaptogens exert a balancing influence on the body; they neither overstimulate nor inhibit normal body function, but rather have a normalizing and tonifying effect. This is completely different from medications that force the body to perform a function even if it is harmful to the body, which is precisely why other medications often have serious side effects while adaptogens do not. Adaptogens are extremely useful in cases of adrenal fatigue, because they normalize several metabolic pathways in the body at once, therefore a single adaptogen can help with both emotional and physical symptoms. Bringing the body back into balance, or homeostasis, is the whole idea behind healing adrenal fatigue, making adaptogens a perfect fit.

When I was finishing chiropractic school, I enrolled in an advanced medical course called, Applied Kinesiology. Applied kinesiology is a series of diagnostic and treatment protocols that are all based on allowing a patient's body to tell the treating physician what is out of balance using a manual muscle test. The basis of applied kinesiology is that the physical, emotional, and biochemistry structure of the body needs to be in balance in order for good health to be achieved. A body out of balance can be restored to balance through various methods involving the nervous system, nutrition, acupuncture meridians (using needles, tapping, laser, and other techniques), chiropractic care, and lifestyle changes. The key point being that proper balance is necessary for good health.

When the body is in balance, you have a perfect equilateral triangle with the physical, emotional, and biochemical components each making up a side of the triangle. When any one of the three sides of the triangle is out of proportion, a person will have symptoms and health issues. Just as it is difficult to change only one side of a triangle, it is difficult to have health issues in only one of the three areas. Adaptogens balance out all three sides of the triangle at the same time. They stimulate the body's systems that need a push and relax the systems that are overworking, resulting in a rebalanced body.

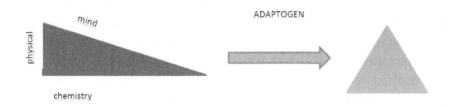

The left side of this figure shows the body out of balance between the mind, physical, and chemistry parts. After an adaptogen is used, the body balances itself out and functions properly. Note how the adaptogen was able to strengthen the weak physical aspect while balancing out the mind and physical sides. That is the true beauty of an adaptogen; it balances both the excited and suppressed systems of the body at the same time.

Adaptogens help balance the body through numerous pathways in response to stress. Their effects on the body can be seen in our moods, physical abilities, and metabolic pathways. They have numerous chemical compounds that work synergistically to improve the body's health on multiple levels, whereas most drugs have a single chemical compound that forces an imbalance in the body, often relieving one problem and starting two others. Medications force the strengthening of only one side of the triangle, causing the other two sides to become imbalanced, and causing additional symptoms.

Adaptogens have been shown to have numerous positive effects on the mind, body, and metabolic pathways, all of which are important to adrenal fatigue sufferers. Some of the ways adaptogens affect the body are:

- Antianxiety

- Antidepressant

- Promote proper body weight

- Increased liver protection and detox function

- Improved mood

- Improved blood sugar handling and balancing

- Decreased alcohol craving

- Decreased sugar cravings

- Improved dietary control

- Improved immune resistance

- Improved antioxidant activity

- Increased energy

- Increased stamina

- Increased libido

- Improved muscle tone

- Increased strength

- Faster recovery from physical exercise

- Improved focus and concentration

- Improved quality of sleep

- Improved motivation and productivity

- Promote a sense of well-being

- Reduced dizziness and vertigo

- Improved gastrointestinal function

The list of positive effects that adaptogens have on the body is impressive and can seem too good to be true. But it's important to remember that adaptogens are, by definition, used to bring the body back into balance on multiple levels at the same time. To achieve their goal of balancing the body, adaptogens need to affect the physical, emotional, and biochemical pathways of the body. This extensive effect is why they are so powerful and useful. You can only be truly healthy when the physical, emotional, and chemical parts of your body are in balance and working well together.

The following is some information about the principal adaptogens that I use in my office. There are two patterns to recognize when reading through the benefits and workings of adaptogens: First, each adaptogen is used to treat multiple symptoms and second, science has revealed that adaptogens are working by affecting the hormones of the adrenal glands.

ASHWAGANDHA (*Withania Somnifera*)

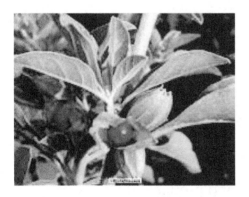

Benefits:

- Increased endurance/anti-fatigue
- Improved sense of well-being
- Anti-inflammatory
- Improved memory and brain function
- Antianxiety

Historical Uses:

Ashwagandha is also known as Indian ginseng or winter cherry. Taken orally, ashwagandha is used for arthritis, anxiety, insomnia, tumors, tuberculosis, chronic liver disease, and as a general tonic. It is also used orally for immunomodulatory effects (regulation of immune system), improving cognitive function, decreasing inflammation, preventing the effects of aging, emaciation, infertility in men and women, menstrual disorders, fibromyalgia, and hiccups. Additionally, ashwagandha is used orally as an aphrodisiac, an emmenagogue (to decrease menstrual flow), and for treating asthma, leukoderma (skin pigmentation disorder), bronchitis, backache, and arthritis.

How it Works:

Research shows that ashwagandha suppresses creation of stress-induced dopamine receptors in the brain. It also appears to reduce stress-induced production of plasma corticosterone (precursor to cortisol and blood lactic acid which is associated with muscle tightness and pain). Ashwagandha seems to have anxiolytic (or relaxation) effects, possibly by acting as a gamma-aminobutyric acid (GABA) mimetic agent.

Safety:

Orally, ashwagandha is well tolerated.

ELEUTHERO ROOT EXTRACT (*Eleutherococcus Senticosus*)

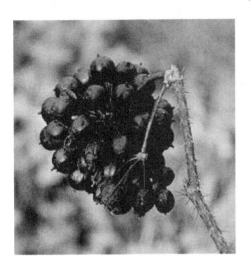

Benefits:

- Increased endurance/anti-fatigue
- Memory/learning improvement
- Anti-inflammatory
- Immunogenic (capable of inducing immune response)
- Antidepressant-like effects

Historical Uses:

Also known as Siberian ginseng, eleuthero root is used orally for normalizing high or low blood pressure, atherosclerosis, pyelonephritis, craniocerebral trauma, rheumatic heart disease, neuroses, insomnia, and increasing work capacity. Other oral uses include Alzheimer's disease, attention deficit-hyperactivity disorder (ADHD), chronic fatigue syndrome, diabetes, fibromyalgia, rheumatoid arthritis, influenza, swine flu, chronic bronchitis, tuberculosis, improving athletic performance, reducing toxicity of chemotherapy, and symptomatic treatment of herpes simplex type II infections. It is also used orally as a general stimulant, diuretic, appetite stimulant, immune system stimulant, and for preventing colds and flu.

How it Works:

Eleuthero root works by stimulating the pituitary-adrenocortical system; it basically helps the brain tell the body how much stress it is under and how best to respond. It has also been shown to prevent viruses from replicating on a DNA-RNA level. Other chemical compounds have been shown to reduce histamine response to help with allergies.

Safety:

Orally, eleuthero root is well tolerated.

LICORICE (*Glycyrrhiza Glabra*)

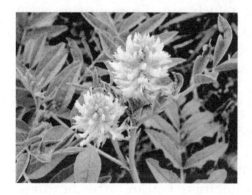

Benefits:

- Relief from gastrointestinal issues
- Anti-stress
- Improved endurance
- Decreased dizziness/vertigo

Historical Uses:

Orally, licorice is used for gastric and duodenal ulcers, sore throat, bronchitis, chronic gastritis, dyspepsia, colic, menopausal symptoms, primary adrenocortical insufficiency, cough, osteoarthritis, osteoporosis, systemic lupus erythematosus (SLE), and for bacterial and viral infections. It is also used orally for cholestatic liver disorders, hypokalemia, hypertonia, malaria, tuberculosis, abscesses, food poisoning, diabetes insipidus, CFS, and contact dermatitis. Additionally, it is used orally to help stimulate adrenal gland function, particularly in patients with a history of long-term corticosteroid use. As a component of the herbal formula shakuyaku-kanzo-to, licorice is used to increase fertility in women with polycystic ovary syndrome. In combination with other herbs, licorice is used to treat prostate cancer and atopic dermatitis (eczema).

How it Works:

Licorice appears to block metabolism of prostaglandins E2 and F2 glycyrrhetinic acids, which are the main causes of gastrointestinal ulcers. It has also been shown to inhibit the conversion of cortisol to inactive cortisone. Cortisol has the effects of increasing energy, salt and water retention, and the ability to deal with stress.

Safety:

Orally, licorice is well tolerated in low dosage. Licorice can change blood pressure, so monitor this if you are on medications.

MAGNOLIA BARK (*Magnolia Biondii*)

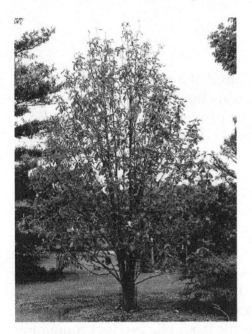

Benefits:

- Angiogenesis inhibitor (inhibits the growth of new blood vessels)
- Antianxiety
- Reduces excessive cortisol
- Helps insomnia

Historical Uses:

Orally, magnolia is used for digestive disorders, constipation, inflammation, and to promote sweating. It is also used for weight loss and obesity, anxiety, stress, depression, fever, headache, stroke, and asthma. Magnolia flower buds are used orally for nasal congestion, runny nose, common cold, sinusitis, allergic rhinitis, headache, and facial dark spots. Topically, magnolia flower buds are used for toothaches. In skin care products, magnolia flower bud extract is used topically as a skin whitener and to minimize or counteract irritant effects of other ingredients.

How it Works:

Magnolol, the bioactive compound of magnolia, suppresses the conversion of cortisol to cortisone by blocking hydroxysteroid dehydrogenase. It increases the production of corticosterone, a glucocorticoid similar to cortisol. This may explain magnolia's use for asthma. Magnolol may also lower cholesterol production. At high doses, magnolia bark seems to have depressant effects on the central nervous system. Honokiol, the bioactive compound of the magnolia bark, seems to inhibit catecholamine secretion. Magnolol and honokiol might enhance cholinergic function, which could be useful in diseases such as Alzheimer's. At high doses, these compounds increase acetylcholine release in the hippocampus of the brain and have a neurotrophic effect, theoretically improving neuronal function. For weight loss, researchers suggest that a specific magnolia product containing a combination of extracts of magnolia plus phellodendron (e.g., Relora®, Next Pharmaceuticals) helps reduce cortisol levels and, therefore, helps to reduce stress. It's theorized that reducing stress will reduce stress-induced eating habits. However, clinical research suggests that this magnolia product does not significantly reduce cortisol levels in overweight women. Magnolia flower buds seem to have uterine stimulating, hypotensive, antifungal, and skeletal-muscle contracting effects. Its constituents, especially magnone, may also have antagonist activity against platelet-activating factors, which might explain its use in nasal congestion and rhinitis.

Magnolia is especially useful for adrenal fatigue patients who are burning themselves out by producing too much cortisol. Often when an adrenal fatigue sufferer doesn't stop producing hormones but instead overproduces hormones, magnolia bark is excellent on this type of patient, because it downregulates the adrenals into balance.

Safety:

Orally, magnolia bark is well tolerated.

RHODIOLA (*Rhodiola Rosea*)

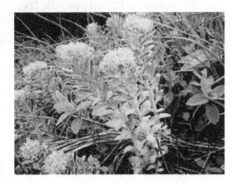

Benefits:

Also known as golden root

- Antidepressant
- Antianxiety
- Increased endurance
- Improved mood
- Improved cognitive function

Historical Uses:

Orally, rhodiola is used for increasing energy, stamina, strength, and mental capacity. It is used for improving athletic performance, improving sexual function, depression, anxiety, cardiac disorders such as arrhythmias, and hyperlipidemia. It is also used for: treating cancer, tuberculosis, and diabetes; preventing cold and flu, swine flu, the effects of aging, and liver damage; improving hearing; strengthening the nervous system; enhancing immunity; and shortening recovery time after prolonged workouts.

How it Works:

Rhodiola works differently than other adaptogens in the fact that it seems to promote endogenous opioid production. Endogenous opioids are the pain-relieving chemical compounds that the brain releases, and they are the most powerful pain modulators in the world. Synthetic opioids are highly addictive for their pain relief and their promotion of a sense of well-being; they include morphine, oxycodone, and methadone. Another mechanism of action for rhodiola is as an MAOI to help with depression. There is also evidence that it promotes the release of norepinephrine to help regulate the sympathetic nervous system. On the physical aspect, it has been shown to increase adenosine triphosphate (ATP), which is used by muscles for energy.

Safety:

Orally, rhodiola is well tolerated.

AMERICAN GINSENG (*Panax Quinquefolius*)

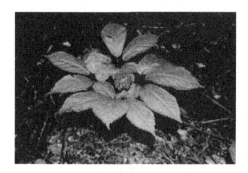

Benefits:

- Improved stress response
- Improved ADHD symptoms
- Helps insomnia

- Helps fibromyalgia
- Improved libido

Historical Uses:

Orally, American ginseng is used to increase resistance to environmental stress, as a general tonic, stimulant, diuretic, and digestive aid. It is also used for anemia, diabetes, insomnia, neurasthenia, gastritis, impotence, fever, hangover symptoms, stimulating immune function, swine flu, human immunodeficiency virus/acquired immunodeficiency syndrome (HIV/AIDS), and ADHD. American ginseng is also used for acute respiratory illness, improving stress resistance, preventing the effects of aging, improving stamina, blood and bleeding disorders, atherosclerosis, loss of appetite, vomiting, colitis, dysentery, breast cancer, insomnia, neuralgia, rheumatism, memory loss, dizziness, headaches, convulsions, fibromyalgia, and disorders of pregnancy and childbirth. In food manufacturing, American ginseng is used in soft drinks and energy drinks. In other manufacturing processes, American ginseng oil and extracts are used in soaps and cosmetics.

How it Works:

American ginseng reduces glucose levels in the blood through increased insulin release and increased cell absorption. It affects the nervous system through the neurotransmitter acetylcholine, which helps with cognitive function. American ginseng changes the physical aspect of the body through the release of nitric oxide, which promotes increased blood flow to muscles and the brain.

Safety:

Orally, American ginseng is well tolerated.

HOLY BASIL (*Ocimum Tenuiflorum*)

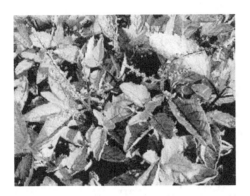

Benefits:

- Anti-inflammatory
- Anti-stress
- Sleep inducing

Historical Uses:

Holy basil is also known asgreen holy basil, hot basil, or Indian basil. Orally, holy basil is used for the common cold, influenza ("the flu"), swine flu, diabetes, asthma, bronchitis, earache, headache, upset stomach, heart disease, fever, viral hepatitis, malaria, stress, and tuberculosis. It is also used for mercury poisoning, to promote longevity, as a mosquito repellent, and as an antidote to snake and scorpion bites.

How it Works:

Holy basil has been shown to inhibit the cyclooxygenase (COX) and lipoxygenase pathways of arachidonic acid metabolism. These are the same pathways that powerful medications like Celebrex® (celecoxib) use to reduce inflammation and pain.

Safety:

Orally, holy basil is well tolerated.

SCHISANDRA CHINENSIS(*Kadsura Chinensis*)

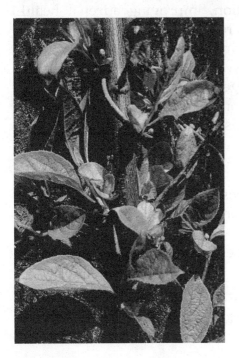

Benefits:

- Improved coordination
- Improved endurance
- Improved concentration

Historical Uses:

Orally, schisandra is used as an adaptogen for increasing resistance to disease and stress, increasing energy, and increasing physical performance and endurance. Schisandra is also taken orally for improving vision, boosting muscular activity, improving cellular energy, for hepatitis, liver protection, preventing premature aging, increasing lifespan, for premenstrual syndrome (PMS), stimulating the immune system, speeding recovery after surgery, protecting against radiation, counteracting the effects of sugar, preventing motion sickness, normalizing blood sugar and blood pressure, reducing high cholesterol, preventing infection, improving adrenal health, and energizing RNA-DNA to rebuild cells. Schisandra is also used to treat coughs, asthma, insomnia, neurasthenia, chronic diarrhea, dysentery, night sweats, spontaneous sweating, involuntary seminal discharge, thirst, impotence, physical exhaustion, excessive urination, depression, irritability, and memory loss. Schisandra fruit is eaten as a food.

How it Works:

The effects of schisandra chinensis on healing the body are well documented. It is considered one of the fifty essential Chinese herbs, but is also a mystery. The mechanism of how it is able to accomplish so many beneficial effects is not known at this time.

Safety:

Orally, schisandra chinensis is well tolerated.

Glandular Supplements: The Master Adaptogens

Glandular supplements (bovine or porcine adrenal supplements) are the most controversial adaptogen and, I think, the most important. Bovine is Latin for "of or relating to the ox or cow," and porcine is Latin for "of or relating to the pig." Bovine or porcine adrenal supplements are made from the adrenal glands of cows or pigs. Glandular supplementation is one of the oldest forms of medicine and is still widely used today. While most of today's medications are derived in labs and chemical factories, many are still animal based. The reason that so many medications are still derived from animal sources is because they are effective, and no good substitutes have been found. The human body was designed to be nourished and healed naturally by the environment. Fruits, vegetables, water, and even animals are a part of that process.

The use of animal hormones, or glandulars, may seem a little odd, but it is actually very common in medicine and is used by tens of millions of Americans every day. The following FDA approved medications are derived from animals:

- Heparin, a blood thinner, is made from pig intestine

- Premarin®, an estrogen replacement drug, is made from horse urine

- Hylaform®, an injectable medication for arthritis, is made from rooster combs

- Pig pancreas is used in tablet form for cystic fibrosis patients

- Magnesium stearate, a filler in medications and a nutritional supplement, is cow-based

- Armour Thyroid®, for hypothyroidism, is made from the thyroid gland of a pig

- Lovaza®, an omega-3 fish oil, is used for cardiac disease

The gel caps used to encase most medications and nutritional supplements are almost always animal-based. The mechanism of how animal glandulars work on the body is more controversial than their actual use as a nutritional supplement.

Physicians and researchers like to know—or pretend they know—how medications affect the body, but the truth is that often a drug is found to work, while the mechanism is never known. The most blatant example of this is statin drugs used to lower cholesterol. It is commonly thought that the "benefits"* of statin drugs come from the lowering of bad cholesterol, but this does not fit the data. Twenty years after statins were first introduced, new research shows that their benefits come from a poorly understood chemical pathway that, when stimulated, reduces arterial inflammation. There has always been a double standard when it comes to drugs versus nutritional supplements. The drug manufactures promote the safety and science behind their medications, only to have their miracle drug of today become the horrific news headline of tomorrow.

Health Note: I used "benefits,"because I do not see any real benefit for the use of statins. The following figures are based on the research provided by Merck & Co. on the best-selling statin, Lipitor® (atorvastatin). If statins were used only for people with a high risk of a cardiac event, it would benefit only 1 percent of that group over a thirty-nine-month period. To save every life, the medication alone would cost roughly five hundred thousand dollars, and if physician appointments, lab testing, and treatment for side effects were also calculated in, the actual cost would be several time higher. It is estimated that 16 percent of all users will have a serious side effect, including muscle weakness, muscle wasting, dementia, and cancer. When you expand the use of statins to the general public, whose only risk is high cholesterol, the cost of saving a life is more than two point five million dollars. A better return on our healthcare dollars would be seen if that money was used for nutritional supplements, nutritional counseling, gym memberships, and weight-loss classes.

There are many theories about how glandular supplements work on the body. Many traditional physicians believe that they do nothing, may be dangerous, and should be removed from the market. Some think that glandular supplements contain a small amount of the hormones, and when taken, they directly increase the hormone levels of the person. Others think that they act as a stimulant to the intended gland and increase its function. Having had more than twenty years of experience using glandular supplements, I have a better idea of how they benefit the body.

The theory of the first group (usually traditional physicians and researchers) — who believe that glandular based nutritional supplements do nothing, may be dangerous, and should be removed from the market — is the easiest to discredit. Their own standards and methods prove them wrong. The FDA has already approved several different glandulars as medications, which proves that there is some value and safety in glandular nutritional supplements. The most commonly used FDA glandular is Armour Thyroid®, which is used for hypothyroidism. It has been taken for decades by millions of Americans with excellent results. It stands to reason that if one animal glandular can be effective, others may be as well. The safety of glandular supplements is beyond reproach, because they have been used for hundreds of years without a single incident. The controversy about adrenal glandulars is compounded by the fact that traditional medicine doesn't even recognize adrenal fatigue. If a condition is not acknowledged, the cure for that condition is certainly not going to be recognized or even tested. Adrenal glandular supplementsare safe and effective, and will be around for a long time to come.

The idea that adrenal glandular supplements supply small amounts of hormones has merit but does not account for their benefits. An adrenal glandular supplement would contain whatever hormones were in the animal's adrenal glands when it was being processed. This amount would be exceedingly small, because the adrenals do not store large amounts of hormones, and the size of the supplement is a fraction of a percent of the glands'total weight. I believe that there is an insufficient quantity of these hormones in adrenal glandulars to account for their powerful benefits.

The concept that adrenal glandular supplements act as a direct stimulant to the adrenals also holds value. New research has shown that the mind and body begin to react to foods, medications, and nutritional supplements the moment they touch your mouth. There is even evidence that the reaction process begins as soon as you smell or touch specific substances, like the gag reflex that occurs when you smell sour milk or the immediate effect of taking nitroglycerin tablets sublingually (under the tongue) to stop a cardiac event. The stimulating effect from the adrenal glandular supplements is involved in the benefits of their use, but I do not believe it to be the main reason they are so effective. My hesitation in accepting this idea stems from the fact that adrenal fatigue is marked by the weakening of the adrenal glands and their inability to respond to stimuli. The weak stimuli from a nutritional supplement would be insufficient to create a positive reaction from the weakened adrenal glands and would not promote their healing but rather their further decline. It is the adrenal glands' failure to react to emotional, physical, or chemical stressors that is the cornerstone of the whole diagnosis of adrenal fatigue.

So how do adrenal glandulars provide such dramatic results for adrenal fatigue sufferers? The answer is simple supply and demand. The adrenal glandular supplements supply the fatigued adrenal glands with the exact nutrients they need to rebuild and rejuvenate themselves. Let me give you an example.

You are building two houses. For the first house, you go to the store and pick up supplies. Your truck only carries so many supplies, so you make a trip, do a little work, then go back to the store before returning to the house again to do a little more work. You repeat this process until the house is done. This is tiresome and wastes a lot of energy. The problem is that you are always waiting on supplies to build your house.

For the second house, all the supplies you may possibly need are delivered to you. With your abundant supplies, you can start and continue to build the house with less overall effort and fatigue, and accomplish the task much faster.

While using adrenal glandular supplements gives you a little bit of the needed hormones and may gently stimulate your system, the true benefit comes from supplying the adrenal glands with all the building blocks for recovery, allowing them to immediately start producing much-needed hormones. This method of action would explain: 1) why adrenal glandulars have a nearly immediate effect on levels of energy, pain, and emotions felt by adrenal fatigue patients; and 2) why they provide long-term benefits for rebuilding the chemical, physical, and emotional components of the body.

Adaptogens, as a group, are the most powerful nutritional supplements to help rebuild the fatigued adrenal glands. When used properly, adrenal fatigue sufferers can feel almost immediate relief and rebuild their systems in little time. While adaptogens are poorly understood in the United States, they have been an important medicinal product in China, India, Russia, and Europe for decades, if not centuries.

Other Key Nutrients to Help with Adrenal Fatigue

There are dozens of nutritional supplements that will help a person recover from adrenal fatigue. The following is a list of just a few of the most important ones, along with an explanation of why each is a key to recovery. Fortunately, many of these nutrients can be provided by the alkaline diet and all of its benefits.

4-AMINO-3-PHENYLBUTYRIC ACID (PHENIBUT)

Phenibut is a GABA derivative. It is a major stimulant to GABA receptors in the brain and reduces the excitatory neurotransmitter phenylethylamine(PEA). Unlike traditional oral GABA nutritional supplements, phenibut has the ability to cross the protective blood-brain barrier and immediately affect our moods. Phenibut provides a very calming and relaxing effect almost immediately upon use and helps promote sleep. It is nonaddictive and helps to restore reduced GABA levels in the body. I like to call it "nature's Xanax®".

L-TRYPTOPHAN

L-tryptophan, which converts to 5-Hydroxytryptophan (5-HTP), is an amino acid used in the synthesis of the neurotransmitter serotonin. 5-HTP is easily absorbed through the gastrointestinal tract and passes through the blood-brain barrier. Oral intake increases serotonin production and levels, which is very calming and helps when dealing with stress.

L-TYROSINE

L-tyrosine is converted into the catecholamine neurotransmitters dopamine, norepinephrine, and epinephrine. Catecholamines are important stimulating neurotransmitters utilized to help the body respond to and recover from stress. They are also significant in balancing the sympathetic nervous system.

L-ARGININE

L-arginine is an amino acid that helps the autonomic nervous system switch between an excited and a relaxed state. It is essential, because it is part of the on-off mechanism of the nervous system.

EPIGALLOCATECHIN GALLATE (EGCG)

EGCG is an active component of green tea. It is an inhibitor of the breakdown of the catecholamine neurotransmitters that excite the nervous system. EGCG has been touted as a weight-loss product for years. The biochemistry behind its success is its ability to keep the body in a stimulated state, burning more calories.

HUPERZIA SERRATA

Huperzia serrata is an herb that prevents the breakdown of the neurotransmitter acetylcholine. Increased acetylcholine helps improve the immune system, cognitive function, and motor function. This product is important for patients with ADHD, fatigue, dementia, and malaise.

MAGNESIUM

Magnesium is a common nutritional supplement. In numerous studies, it has been shown to reduce brain excitability. It stimulates the same receptors as GABA and prevents or reduces the stimulating effect of glutamate.

MELATONIN

Melatonin is a natural hormone produced by our bodies and by plants. Melatonin is well known for its effects on the sleep-wake cycle.

MUCUNA COCHINCHINESIS

Mucuna cochinchinensis is an herbal source of L-3,4-dihydroxyphenylalanine (L-DOPA) which converts into dopamine. Dopamine is a major excitatory neurotransmitter for the nervous system and is involved in fighting depression and Parkinson's disease.

PHOSPHATIDYLSERINE

Phosphatidylserine is important to reestablishing communication along the hypothalamus-pituitary-adrenal (HPA) axis. The HPA axis becomes desensitized to stress and inactive after an acute trauma or prolonged stress. Reestablishing normal function of the HPA axis is key to healing adrenal fatigue, PTSD, CFS, anxiety, and depression.

TAURINE

Taurine is an important amino acid involved in relaxation. It works by binding to GABA receptors to promote relaxation. It also helps to increase the synthesis of GABA, reduce the breakdown of GABA, and keep GABA working longer as a neurotransmitter. Taurine is a major factor in promoting the sense of calmness in the mind and body.

Note of Interest: Taurine is a major component in most high-caffeine energy drinks. Without taurine, the high levels of caffeine and other stimulants would overwhelm the nervous system and cause panic attacks and heart palpitations.

THEANINE

Theanine is an amino acid naturally found in green tea and is used to calm the mind and body. It works by calming an overstimulated nervous system by blocking glutamate receptors. Glutamate is a stimulating neurotransmitter, and by blocking its receptors, theanine prevents continued stimulation and promotes a calming effect.

VITAMIN B

The group of B vitamins is a vital nutritional factor in adrenal function. Nearly every biochemical pathway involving the adrenal glands requires several different B vitamins.

Nutritional supplementation for adrenal fatigue involves a combination of proper diet, amino acids, vitamins, and herbs. While the task of figuring out which supplements to take may seem daunting, it is not that complex. Most nutritional supplements, like adaptogens, are designed to bring homeostasis and good health to the body. Rarely does your symptomatic relief or general health rely on you picking the exactly-correct nutrient. Natural nutritional supplements usually contain a variety of ingredients and compounds, and together they will help to restore balance and health to your body.

Interesting Note: Drug companies are obsessed with finding the one key chemical compound in a plant that causes a positive reaction. This single compound can then be patented and made into a drug. The true reason why most herbal or nutritional supplements work so well is that they have multiple chemical compounds that work synergistically to create a greater and better-rounded effect then any single compound. For example, red yeast rice contains several chemical compounds, including some lovastatin, the main ingredient in Merck & Co.'s statin drug,Mevacor®.When compared against each other, red yeast rice was less expensive, saved more lives, reduced more cardiac events, and had fewer side effects than its pharmaceutical counterpart.

The body is designed to heal itself with what is found in nature. All you need to do is help it along with a good diet, proper physical activity, and some general nutritional supplements. The body will do the rest.

Physical Treatments to Heal Adrenal Fatigue

The vast majority of people suffering with adrenal fatigue are plagued with physical symptoms. There are a wide range of symptoms that occur with adrenal fatigue, and often the symptoms do not seem related and can change quickly. The one common factor that almost all adrenal fatigue sufferers have in common is a physical pain or discomfort that is not relieved fully, no matter what type of care they receive.

The physical pain that accompanies adrenal fatigue is in direct response to the inability of the patient's body to handle the physical, emotional, and/or chemical stress from which they suffer. One of the first problems to occur in adrenal fatigue is ligament laxity. Ligament laxity is when the ligaments, tendons, muscles, and joints are too loose to keep a joint stabilized. This instability leads to several problems, including muscle strain, ligament and tendon sprain, and joint inflammation. Continued joint inflammation can then turn into arthritic changes, tendon tears, and more serious conditions. Interestingly, when you address adrenal fatigue, many of the "untreatable"ailments like arthritis, torn ligaments, and chronic pains will abate. This miraculous recovery is due to the increased stability in the associated joint.

Physical pain is usually what will bring an adrenal fatigue sufferer to the doctor, but it is often misdiagnosed. This first missed opportunity to address adrenal fatigue leads to many more misdiagnoses as the condition worsens and the symptoms change. The variety of physical complaints, the fact that the pains are constantly changing, and the stress from the pains all usually lead physicians to recommend antidepressant or antianxiety medications. These types of medications may relieve the physical pain for the moment, but as the body adapts to the medication, the pain returns.

The following is a partial list of physical complaints often linked to adrenal fatigue. When reading the list, you will probably notice that you have or have recently had several of these conditions:

- Headaches

- Dizziness

- Cigarette, sugar, carbohydrate, and/or alcohol cravings

- Vertigo

- Temporomandibular joint (TMJ) pains

- Tendonitis

- Bursitis

- Blurry vision

- Muscle spasms

- Trigger points

- Gastrointestinal issues (such as constipation or diarrhea)

- Fatigue (especially first thing in the morning, improving throughout the day)

- Decreased endurance

- Weight gain

- Increased belly fat

- Pain, especially in the back (increased with deep breaths)

- Pain hours afteror the next day afterexercise, but not usually with exercise

- Insomnia

- Premenstrual symptoms

- Poor sexual function and desire

- Chronic sprains and strains

- Common physical complaints (misdiagnosis for adrenal fatigue included)

- Fibromyalgia

- Orthostatic hypotension

- Chronic fatigue syndrome (CFS)

- Pain syndrome

- Postural orthostatic tachycardia syndrome (POTS)

- Cluster headaches

- Migraines

Adrenal fatigue sufferers usually have so many physical complaints that they often state, "I am just falling apart."The fact that so many varied things are wrong with a patient is a great sign that they have adrenal fatigue. These patients are the best to treat, because they do so well with my adrenal fatigue healing program.

While I believe that the nutritional aspect of this program provides the greatest benefit to adrenal fatigue sufferers, there still is a need to address some complaints with physical care. Nutrition will be able to rebuild the adrenals and the body, but certain conditions need to be treated hands on. That is why treatments offered in my practice often combine many of the following therapies:

ORIENTAL MEDICINE

Americans associate Oriental medicine with acupuncture and needles, but Oriental medicine is actually based on the flow of qi (pronounced "chee") through meridians that surround the body. Qi, in its simplest explanation, is the body's energy force, and the meridians are the pathways the qi must travel to energize and heal the body. Any disruption in the flow of the body's qi can lead to physical, emotional, or biochemical imbalance and symptoms.

The body's qi can be balanced and helped along the meridians in a number of different ways. While acupuncture is what most Americans think of when Oriental medicine is discussed, there are other ways to affect the strength and flow of qi, including nutrition, Oriental massages, acupressure, moxibustion, and alarm-point stimulation with tapping.

Maintaining balance of the flow and strength of your body's qi is important to overall health, because it will promote healing on a physical, mental, and biochemical level.

APPLIED KINESIOLOGY

Applied kinesiology is a diagnostic and treatment program that is utilized by physicians with advanced training. The system is based on how the body changes in relation to different stimuli. While applied kinesiology is only practiced by a select few physicians in the United States, it is a medical specialty in Europe, just like being an internist or a cardiologist.

Applied kinesiology is extremely effective, because it can be used to diagnose emotional, physical, and biochemical dysfunctions, with given methods to treat any detected dysfunctions. Treatment methods include physical mobilization of joints and muscles, stimulating acupuncture meridians, nutrition, craniopathy, massage, and even a form of cognitive therapy. A good applied kinesiologist can treat almost all health conditions in a safe and effective manner. I would strongly recommend finding a local applied kinesiologist to help guide you through your adrenal fatigue healing process. Applied kinesiology is the ideal treatment method for adrenal fatigue, because it is designed to look at the physical, emotional, and biochemical aspects of all health conditions.

NEURO EMOTIONAL TECHNIQUE (NET)

NET is a combination of chiropractic, nutrition, acupuncture, and stress visualization. NET is practiced by physicians and is a way to link the mind and body together. Often patients will have emotional stress that causes physical pain or physical pain that causes emotional stress. NET allows for the two to be separated and healed.

NET allows the patient to visualize their pain, touch their pain, or think about their stress or stressors and then be desensitized. The desensitization to the aggravating factors is done by stimulating treatment points along the qi meridians and then strengthened using nutritional supplements. I find NET to be a quick and effective way to eliminate pain and stress brought on by negative thoughts and situations.

Note: NET is often done by physicians who practice applied kinesiology.

YOGA

Yoga is a system of poses designed to stimulate the body's musculoskeletal system and relax the mind. It is an excellent exercise, because it actively involves the mind and body in the same event. The deep breathing involved in yoga is excellent for naturally stimulating a nerve cluster found behind the chest wall that promotes relaxation.

I do recommend that if you start a yoga program, you start off slowly. The low impact of yoga is excellent for adrenal fatigue patients, but too vigorous of a stretch can cause inflammation and pain. I recommend that you stretch just until you feel a light tug, and then hold. Do not try to stretch to the end range. Adrenal fatigue sufferers tend to have very loose ligaments, tendons, and joints, which is why they have so much pain. Too vigorous of a stretch can severely aggravate your condition.

CRANIAL ELECTRICAL STIMULATION (CES)

CES is a rarely-used but extremely effective treatment to help relieve physical pain and emotional stress. This therapy is very simple and can be done at home on a regular basis. CES is provided by a battery-powered, phone-sized device. The device is connected to your body by ear clips. CES works by sending an electric wave in an alpha form from one ear to the other. You do not feel — or barely feel — the wave. Alpha waves stimulate the brain's own alpha waves in order to produce endorphins.

Research has shown that people with PTSD, fibromyalgia, or chronic stress produce fewer alpha waves and thus fewer endorphins. The reduction in endorphins from the lack of alpha waves leads to anxiety, insomnia, and pain. Endorphins are natural opiates that relax a person and reduce pain. I recommend CES devices to my patients, because they not only provide relief very quickly, but also help to retrain the brain to produce more alpha waves, and thus endorphins, on its own. Unlike medications that become less effective with time, CES retrains the brain to handle stress and pain more efficiently and becomes more effective with continued use.

Emotional Therapies to Heal Adrenal Fatigue

Adrenal fatigue very often follows a traumatic emotional event such as a death, a bad accident, or a divorce. The benefits of a little talk time with a psychotherapist, or at least a friend, are invaluable to healing adrenal fatigue. While I often recommend a patient see a psychotherapist if they feel overwhelmed, more often they have been seeing one for years before finding me. Adrenal fatigue is found almost exclusively in motivated and driven people, and many of them are uncomfortable with the idea of seeing a psychotherapist. The following are several options available either for those who prefer not to see a psychotherapist or to be used in combination with psychotherapy:

COGNITIVE BEHAVIORAL THERAPY (CBT)

CBT is based on the idea that anxiety and depression may be out of the control of those affected. It first trains the sufferer to notice the early warning signs of an impending attack. Then, it teaches the sufferer to implement coping mechanisms, such as deep breathing, to preventthe attack before it happens. CBT has been shown to be more effective than traditional talk therapy for many conditions.

BIOFEEDBACK

Biofeedback, by definition, is a process that enables an individual to learn how to change physiological activity for the purposes of improving health and performance. Precise instruments measure physiological activity, such as brainwaves, heart function, breathing, muscle activity, and skin temperature. These instruments rapidly and accurately feed back information to the user. The presentation of this information — often in conjunction with changes in thinking, emotions, and behavior — supports desired physiological changes. Over time, these changes can endure without continued use of the biofeedback instrument.

I like to think of biofeedback as a combination of CBT and CES. As with CBT, you are training yourself to be more aware of when your mind and body are becoming overwhelmed, and then applying methods in which you were trained, such as deep breathing, to restore normal physiological patterns. Restoring normal physiological patterns is also how the CES unit affects the mind and body.

NEURO EMOTIONAL TECHNIQUE (NET)
CRANIAL ELECTRICAL STIMULATION (CES)

Previously covered under Physical Treatments, NET and CES are also emotional therapies.

Synergistic Healing

Adrenal fatigue involves the emotional, physical, and biochemical aspects of the body. The only way to properly heal from adrenal fatigue is to make sure that all three facets are supported, so that homeostasis is restored. Fortunately, the body is designed to rebuild and heal itself with just a little extra help. The nutritional supplements listed in this chapter will help reduce your physical pain, relieve your emotional stress, and restore your body's natural chemical balance. The physical treatments mentioned will help reduce physical pain, mental stress, and the toxins in your system in order to regain chemical balance. The emotional techniques relieve stress on the chemical pathways in your nervous system and provide relief from physical pain while stabilizing your overall anxiety and mood. The whole program is designed to work synergistically.

Matthew

Before going to see Dr. Zodkoy, my son, Matthew, was suffering with debilitating symptoms. His most prevalent symptom was severe germophobia. He had a terrible fear of getting germs, so he would wash his hands excessively. He also believed that his sister was the root of the issue, so he would avoid her and anything she touched. If he had to walk where she had walked — for instance, up the stairs — he would cover himself in a sheet.

This was very limiting in the home and at school too, as his sister also attended the same school. He was very nervous and wouldn't take a shower at school. He was afraid that his sister had been in the classroom that he was in, so he would avoid sitting on the chair or would sit on his heels so that he didn't actually touch the chair.

My wife and I tried taking him to a psychiatrist, who suggested Zoloft® (sertraline). This medication took the edge off of the problem but did not solve it.

Once we began seeing Dr. Zodkoy, Matthew felt better very quickly. In just two weeks, he was 50 percent better. Dr. Zodkoy put him on supplements and did alternative therapies with him to help him adjust.

Afterward, he was just a happier kid who could walk through the hallways without concern. He would also sit on the couch without a sheet under him — something he would never have done before!

Dr. Zodkoy exuded confidence and was very understanding and caring. A year later, Matthew is doing much better! We can't thank Dr. Zodkoy enough!

Chapter Seven
Using an Alkaline Diet
to Beat Adrenal Fatigue

Dr. Howard Cohn, DC
Founder and Director, Cohn Health Institute, CHI
(www.CohnHealthInstitute.com)
Co-Founder and Chief Product Officer, SevenPoint2,
The Alkaline Company (www.SevenPoint2.com)

"Life is really simple,
but men insist on making it complicated."
– Confucius, 551–479 BC

Why Adopt an Alkaline Diet?

After working with thousands of patients over two decades on their diet and nutrition, there is one thing that I have observed time and time again: Those who can successfully adopt an alkaline diet get better and recover faster than those who do not, regardless of the condition. It is really that simple. The problem is that it is not always easy. It can be very time consuming and is not always cost effective. The biggest problem of all is that it is definitely *not* palatable.

In this chapter, we will discuss the history and efficacy of the alkaline diet, measuring pH and why it is important, and new and effective strategies that allow everyone to attain and maintain an alkaline lifestyle.

What is an Alkaline Diet?

So what actually *is* an alkaline diet? Simply put, the foods that we eat each and every day fall into one of two categories: they are either acid-forming or alkaline-forming foods. Generally, acid-forming foods are traditionally associated with increasing inflammation throughout the body, and inflammation is associated with most health challenges that people suffer from today. Alkaline-forming foods are traditionally more oxygenating foods and are more likely to assist in recovery and maintenance of good health.

So which foods are acidic, and which are alkaline? Okay, get ready, because here comes the bad news. Meat, chicken, fish, cheese, milk, bread, pasta, coffee, beer, wine, soda, and ice cream are all examples of acidic foods. (See Figure A for a more complete listing of acidifying foods.) Examples of alkaline foods include broccoli, kale, chard, cabbage, wheatgrass, and barley grass. (See Figure B for a more complete listing of alkalizing foods.)

Acidifying Foods					
Corn	Rye	Spelt	Oatmeal	Bread	Pasta
Chocolate	Fish	Beef	Chicken	Pork	Milk
Cheese	Yogurt	Wheat	Butter	Beer	Wine
Coffee	Sugar	Ketchup	Mustard	Alcohol	Lamb
Duck	Lard	Shellfish	Nuts	Eggs	French fries
Pizza	Tacos	Hamburgers	Soy	Tap water	Turkey
Popcorn	Cake	Candy	Table salt	Jam	Jelly
Pickles	Pies	Beans	Donuts	Chickpeas	Bran
Bison	Cranberries	Bacon	Sausage	Artificial sweeteners	Bagels

Figure A

Alkalizing Foods					
Lettuce	Broccoli	Beets	Chard	Collard greens	Wheatgrass
Oat grass	Barley grass	Alfalfa	Kale	Celery	Cauliflower
Eggplant	Avocado	Coconut	Cherries	Blackberries	Apples
Grapes	Grapefruit	Raspberries	Strawberries	Watermelon	Garlic
Onions	Raisins	Ginger	Ghee	Lemons	Limes
Oranges	Pineapples	Pears	Peaches	Mango	Papaya
Cantaloupe	Honeydew	Banana	Apricot	Potato	Peppers
Quinoa	Pumpkin	Sauerkraut	Mushrooms	Parsnip	Radishes
Sea salt	Parsley	Kelp	Nori	Sprouts	Squash
Green beans	Turnips	Carrots	Brussels sprouts	Mustard greens	Endive
Zucchini	Yams	Okra			

Figure B

Why Don't Most People Eat an Alkaline Diet?

These examples should give you a pretty good understanding of why it is so hard for people to eat an alkaline diet. We are ruled by our palates. If broccoli tasted as good as an ice cream sundae, then everyone would want to eat an alkaline diet. Most people remember the first time they tried wheatgrass, because it is usually also the last time they had it. The commentary usually goes something like this:

"It tasted like I just licked the bottom of my lawnmower. I'm never doing that again."

And that's the end of their alkaline diet.

Most of us end up subscribing to a philosophy similar to that of Mark Twain, who I believe once said, "I know I would live ten years longer if I quit smoking, but that would be ten years without cigarettes."

History of the Alkaline Diet

Although the alkaline diet has become quite popular over the past few years, it is not a new concept. French surgeon and biologist, Dr. Alexis Carrel, winner of the 1912 Nobel Prize in Physiology or Medicine, was quoted as saying, "The human cell is immortal, as long as we maintain the alkaline fluids that it is bathed in."

In 1933, Dr. William Howard Hay, originator of the concept of food combining said, "Now we depart from health in just the proportion to which we have allowed our alkalis to be dissipated by introduction of acid-forming food in too great amount... It may seem strange to say that all disease is the same thing, no matter what its myriad modes of expression, but it is verily so."

Perhaps the most straightforward statement on the subject is from Arthur Guyton, MD, author of the *Textbook of Medical Physiology*. In his definitive textbook, Dr. Guyton states, "The first step to maintaining health is to alkalize the body. The cells of a healthy body are alkaline while the cells of a diseased body are acidic. Since our bodies do not manufacture alkalinity, we must supply the alkalinity from an outside source to keep us from being acidic and dying."

Measuring pH

The abbreviation pH stands for potential of hydrogen. Saliva and urine pH are measured using litmus paper. A scale of 1 to 14 is used to measure pH, with 1 being most acidic, 7 being neutral pH, and 14 being most alkaline (see Figure C). Blood pH is usually measured in a hospital using a specific pH test called an arterial blood gas (ABG). Blood pH runs ideally at 7.365 and does not vary up or down by even a decimal point unless the body is in an acute health-care crisis. It may seem that the difference between, for example, 6.2 and 7.2 is a small thing, because it is just a point, but this is a big thing since the pH scale is logarithmic. This means that if you test at 6.2, you're actually ten times more acidic than if you're testing at 7.2. If you're testing at 5.2, then you're a hundred times more acidic than at 7.2! That's a big deal when it comes to your health.

For our purposes, we can get a lot of information about the state of health of our internal body systems by regularly checking our saliva and urinary pH. Although there are a variety of reasons why pH can vary up or down, as a general rule, we are at our healthiest when the pH of our tissues runs consistently on the slightly alkaline side.

pH Scale

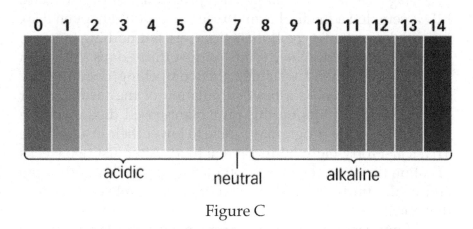

Figure C

Where We Are Now

So where are we today as a nation? Where have our overly acidic diets gotten us? Some sources are now reporting that four out of five Americans will die of cancer, heart disease, or stroke. Diabetes is quickly becoming an epidemic, with sixty-nine percent of the population considered overweight or obese. We are not getting any younger either, since every six seconds, one of our over seventy-six million baby boomers turns fifty years old. In the March, 2005 issue of the *New England Journal of Medicine,* Dr. David S. Ludwig, director of the obesity program at Children's Hospital Boston, states, "Obesity is such that this generation of children could be the first, basically in the history of the United States, to live less healthful and shorter lives than their parents." According to the World Health Organization (WHO), by 2015, approximately two point three billion adults worldwide will be overweight, with more than seven hundred million obese. Talk about some heavy stress on the adrenals!

Pretty scary stuff, huh? Well, it doesn't have to be. Just take a look at a documentary that was done not long ago called, *Simply Raw: Reversing Diabetes in 30 Days*. In this program, Gabriel Cousens, MD assembled a medical team to see what would happen if six insulin-dependent, type II diabetics were fed nothing but raw, green, plant-based, whole foods for just thirty days. Although I highly recommend watching this compelling documentary in its entirety, here is a brief summation of the results. After just forty-eight hours on this raw, plant-based diet, everyone who followed the program was able to lower their insulin dose. That's just forty-eight hours on real food! After just two weeks of eating this way, they were completely off insulin, and by the end of the thirty days, they were medically released as non-diabetic.It really is that simple. The only problem is that the diet is not easy to do. One participant was quoted as saying something to the effect of they would rather be dead than to have to spend their life having to eat this way. Herein lies the human condition. As the legendary Jim Henson Muppets character, Kermit the Frog, once put it, "It's not easy being green."

Looking at adopting an alkaline diet is not a fad; it has become a necessity. Diabetes and obesity are just the tip of the iceberg. Here is a partial list of conditions that have been associated with chronic acidosis:

- Headaches and migraines
- Bladder conditions
- Kidney stones
- Immune deficiency
- Lack of energy and fatigue
- Acne
- Dry skin
- Hyperactivity

- Dizziness
- Panic attacks
- Joint pain
- Depressive tendencies
- Cardiovascular damage
- Food allergies
- Chemical sensitivities
- Hair loss
- Weak nails
- Slow digestion and elimination
- Yeast or fungal overgrowth
- Hormonal problems
- Premature aging
- Loose and painful teeth
- Excess stomach acid
- Lack of drive, joy, and enthusiasm
- Low body temperature
- Insomnia
- Viral and bacterial infections
- Asthma
- Learning disabilities
- Loss of memory and concentration
- Ulcers
- Osteoporosis
- Arthritis
- Colitis
- Tendonitis
- And pretty much everything else that ends with an "itis"

Does that list sound like anyone you know?

Benefits of Raw Green Foods

So what makes these raw green foods so special? Well, there are many things, but one element that sticks out in particular is chlorophyll, the molecule that makes green plants green and the integral part of the plant that helps to create oxygen (without which we would all perish, so it's pretty important). The list of health benefits from chlorophyll alone is enough to take up a whole page in this text. It is also almost identical in its structure to the hemoglobin molecule in human blood (see Figure D).

Hemoglobin Molecule and Chlorophyll Molecule

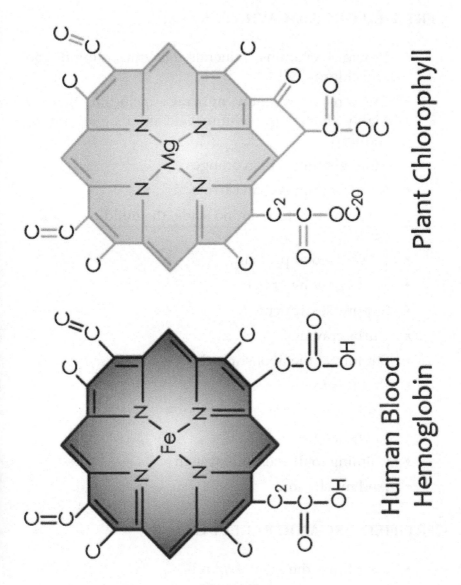

Figure D

Here are some examples of just a handful of these green foods and what makes them special:

CERTIFIED ORGANIC WHATGRASS:

- Provides vitamins, minerals, enzymes, amino acids, and chlorophyll
- Contains over ninety minerals, including the most highly alkaline (potassium, calcium, magnesium, and sodium)
- More vitamin C than oranges
- More vitamin A than carrots
- Contains nineteen amino acids, the building blocks to protein
- Lowers blood pressure
- Slows graying of hair
- Suppresses appetite
- Curbs cravings
- Stimulates metabolism and circulation
- Reduces tooth decay
- Anti-inflammatory
- Energizing
- Calming to the nervous system
- And much more

CERTIFIED ORGANIC BARLEY GRASS:

- Four times the calcium of milk
- At least five times the iron of spinach
- As much protein, per ounce, as steak
- Loaded with every essential amino acid

- Twenty-three percent of barley grass is digestible protein
- Packed with thirteen vitamins and twelve minerals
- A true "superfood"

CERTIFIED ORGANIC OAT GRASS:

- Great source of beta carotene, vitamins C and K, folic acid, B vitamins, protein, fiber, and calcium
- Aids in heart health and helps to lower cholesterol
- Helps to increase energy and stamina
- Has been shown to help lower blood sugar
- Has been consumed as a food by humans since prehistoric times

CERTIFIED ORGANIC KALE:

- Potent antioxidant
- Loaded with fiber
- Contains omega-3 fatty acids
- Curbs appetite
- Anti-inflammatory
- Rich in calcium, copper, iron, and manganese
- Per calorie, kale has more calcium than milk
- Naturally detoxifying

CERTIFIED ORGANIC SPINACH:

- High in fiber
- Shown to effectively lower blood pressure
- Loaded with antioxidants, including vitamins C, E,

and beta-carotene, as well as lutein and zeaxanthin, which protect the eyes from cataracts and age-related macular degeneration

- Boosts immunity
- Helps build strong bones
- Contains omega-3 fatty acids
- Natural anti-inflammatory

CERTIFIED ORGANIC PARSLEY:

- Packed with antioxidants, especially vitamins A and C
- Potent anti-inflammatory
- Helps support your immune system
- Helps the heart by controlling homocysteine levels
- Cultivated for over two thousand years
- The world's most popular herb

CERTIFIED ORGANIC CABBAGE:

- Loaded with folic acid, vitamin C, beta-carotene, vitamin E, and fiber
- Powerful anti-inflammatory
- Rich in iron, sulfur, iodine, calcium, magnesium, and potassium
- Contains sulforaphane, which stimulates the production of glutathione
- Said to promote healthy weight loss

CERTIFIED ORGANIC BROCCOLI:

- Rich in fiber

- High in vitamin C and folic acid

- Great source of potassium

- Rich in vitamin K and calcium to help support healthy bones

- Helps to promote healthy blood pressure

- Contains glucoraphanin, which helps the skin to detoxify and repair itself from sun damage

Note: A word about organic. It is recommended that all foods you consume be organic due to the staggering amounts of pesticides, herbicides, fungicides, and countless other chemicals, toxins, and poisons that have corrupted our air, water, and food supplies. You can minimize exposure to these harmful chemicals by choosing organic as often as possible.

If, for some reason, you still are questioning the absolute necessity of a whole food, plant-based, alkaline diet, then pick yourself up a copy of *The China Study*, by T. Colin Campbell. Subtitled,*The Most Comprehensive Study on Nutrition Ever Conducted*, the book is based on a twenty-year joint project between Cornell University, Oxford University, and the Chinese Academy of Preventive Medicine. The study surveyed the eating habits of sixty-five hundred adults, from all over China and Taiwan, and found a direct correlation between diet and disease.

Okay, so we need to eat this way, but how are we going to do it? If it were easy, everyone would probably be doing it already. After twenty-three years of practice, I've seen less than two percent of my patients change their diets completely, as described by Doctors Cousens and Campbell. So what about the other ninety-eight percent? Are they doomed?

The Easy Way to Go Alkaline

After years of frustration due to lack of compliance, follow-through, and maintenance of an alkaline diet, I decided to find a solution rather than to continue to throw my hands up in disappointment. I worked out a program that anyone and everyone could do, whether young or old, sick or healthy, and even those who hated greens. I helped design a line of products to support and supplement any diet and turn it into an alkaline diet. They are now being produced by SevenPoint2™, The Alkaline Company, and they are becoming a worldwide phenomenon. For the first time in history, it is now simple, easy, cost-effective, and most of all, palatable to be alkaline. Anyone can do it—*even you!*

We call the program, The Seven-Week Alkaline Transformation (www.SevenPoint2Transformation.com). It's *not* another fad diet. It's *not* another brutal workout program. It's real change based on real science and basic human physiology.

trans for ma tion (noun): a seemingly miraculous change in appearance

Most people have, at some time in their lives, tried a diet. While most traditional weight-loss plans can help you lose weight, the biggest challenge is that many times they can make your health worse by causing your body to become too acidic. This, in turn, can cause a major disruption in your metabolism, so even if you do lose weight, you end up gaining it back even faster.

How the Transformation works is simple, and the key is alkalinity. When you eat acidic foods, it can send the body into a fight-or-flight response, causing it to store the excess acid as fat. When you eat alkaline foods, your body tends to emulsify fat (take big fat and turn it into little fat), making it easier for your body to better digest and eliminate. This one fundamental key, coupled with the breakthrough concept of "nutrient timing," is what makes the SevenPoint2 Alkaline Transformation the *only* program of its type to produce *real*, lasting change.

Please Note: It is always important to consult your healthcare provider or physician before starting any new exercise or diet program.

The Seven-Week Alkaline Transformation

BASIC

Take 1 serving of the SevenPoint2 Shake and 1 serving of the SevenPoint2 Greens per day. Replace your SevenPoint2 Shake at lunch with 3.5 ounces of protein source at one of your meals (see Menu Options).

FAST TRACK

Take 2 servings of the SevenPoint2 Shake and 2 servings of the SevenPoint2 Greens per day (one at breakfast and one during your afternoon or evening snack).

Note: One of the Shake portions is used to replace one of the protein sources at lunch or dinner (see Menu Options).

Recommended Food Portions for the Seven-Week Transformation:

During the program: 80 percent alkaline foods and 20 percent acid foods

Maintenance: 60 percent alkaline foods and 40 percent acid foods

Seven-Week Transformation FAST TRACK Menu Options:

DAY ONE

Upon Rising: Take 2-3 SevenPoint2 Recovery tablets with an 8-ounce glass of water

Breakfast: SevenPoint2 Shake and SevenPoint2 Greens

Snack: 10 raw organic almonds and a small piece of fruit

Lunch: SevenPoint2 Shake and spinach salad: 2 cups spinach, ¼ cup mushrooms, ¼ cup cucumber, ¼ cup carrot with 1 tablespoon vinaigrette dressing

Snack: 2-3 SevenPoint2 Green caps andcelery or apples with 1 tablespoon almond or sunflower seed butter

Dinner: 3-5 ounces organic chicken breast, ½ cup broiled beets, and ½ cup steamed broccoli

Snack (optional): Small peach, halved and baked with 1 teaspoon vanilla and (optional) sprinkle of cinnamon

At Bedtime: Take 4 SevenPoint2 Alkaline Boosters

DAY TWO

Upon Rising: Take 2-3 SevenPoint2 Recovery tablets with an 8-ounce glass of water

Breakfast: SevenPoint2 Shake and SevenPoint2 Greens

Snack: Celery or apples with 1 tablespoon almond or sunflower seed butter

Lunch: SevenPoint2 Shake and veggie wrap: 2 large pieces of lettuce (Butter or Romaine) with carrots, cucumber, onion, and spinach sprinkled inside the leaves, seasoned with 1 tablespoon vinaigrette dressing

Snack: 2-3 SevenPoint2 Green caps andunsweetened yogurt (goat milk, coconut, or almond) with ½ cup fruit, sweetened with stevia or 1 tablespoon maple syrup

Dinner: 3-5 ounces baked wild halibut, seasoned to choice, with 1 cup steamed cauliflower and broccoli mix

Snack (optional): 1 small piece of sliced fruit

At Bedtime: Take 4 SevenPoint2 Alkaline Boosters

DAY THREE

Upon Rising: Take 2-3 SevenPoint2 Recovery tablets with an 8-ounce glass of water

Breakfast: SevenPoint2 Shake and SevenPoint2 Greens

Snack: 1 plain rice cake with a small piece of fruit

Lunch: SevenPoint2 Shake and veggie wrap: 2 large pieces of lettuce (Butter or Romaine) with carrots, cucumber, onion, and spinach sprinkled inside the leaves, seasoned with 1 tablespoon vinaigrette dressing

Snack: 2-3 SevenPoint2 Green caps and½ cup of sliced cucumbers with 2 tablespoons hummus

Dinner: 3-5 ounces grilled wild salmon, seasoned with lemon and garlic, 1 cup of green vegetables of choice, and small dinner salad

Snack (optional): 1 slice of watermelon ½ inch thick

At Bedtime: Take 4 SevenPoint2 Alkaline Boosters

DAY FOUR

Upon Rising: Take 2-3 SevenPoint2 Recovery tablets with an 8-ounce glass of water

Breakfast: SevenPoint2 Shake and SevenPoint2 Greens

Snack: 1 plain rice cake with 1 tablespoon almond or sunflower seed butter

Lunch: SevenPoint2 Shake and 2 cups of grilled seasoned vegetables

Snack: 2-3 SevenPoint2 Green caps andsliced apples with cinnamon sprinkled on top

Dinner: 3-5 ounces grilled bison burger in lettuce wrap with your favorite fresh vegetable fixings (e.g. tomato, onion, pickle), 1 cup steamed asparagus

Snack (optional): Celery or apples with 1 tablespoon almond or sunflower seed butter

At Bedtime: Take 4 SevenPoint2 Alkaline Boosters

DAY FIVE

Upon Rising: Take 2-3 SevenPoint2 Recovery tablets with an 8-ounce glass of water

Breakfast: SevenPoint2 Shake and SevenPoint2 Greens

Snack: Unsweetened yogurt (goat milk, coconut or almond) with 5 crumbled walnuts and 1 tablespoon maple syrup

Lunch: SevenPoint2 Shake and vegetable stir fry: ½ cup each of broccoli, cauliflower, mushrooms, bok choy, and snap peas, sautéed with 1 teaspoon olive oil and 2 tablespoons coconut aminos

Snack: 2-3 SevenPoint2 Green caps and1 piece of fruit

Dinner: Taco salad: 3-5 ounces ground, grass-fed beef or organic ground chicken or turkey, seasoned with no-sugar taco seasoning, placed on top of 2 cups lettuce, sliced onions, ¼ cup chopped tomatoes, ½ small avocado, and 2 tablespoons salsa

Snack (optional): 10 organic almonds and a small piece of fruit

At Bedtime: Take 4 SevenPoint2 Alkaline Boosters

DAY SIX

Upon Rising: Take 2-3 SevenPoint2 Recovery tablets with an 8-ounce glass of water

Breakfast: SevenPoint2 Shake and SevenPoint2 Greens

Snack: ¼ cup raw or roasted unsweetened pumpkin seeds

Lunch: SevenPoint2 Shake and grilled zucchini and asparagus over lettuce, seasoned with your favorite Cajun seasoning

Snack: 2-3 SevenPoint2 Green caps and10 mini organic carrots

Dinner: Taco salad: 3-5 ounces grilled fish of choice with 2 cups mixed grilled vegetables (zucchini, bell peppers, eggplant, asparagus, summer squash)

Snack (optional): 1 cup mixed berries

At Bedtime: Take 4 SevenPoint2 Alkaline Boosters

DAY SEVEN

Upon Rising: Take 2-3 SevenPoint2 Recovery tablets with an 8-ounce glass of water

Breakfast: SevenPoint2 Shake and SevenPoint2 Greens

Snack: 10 raw organic walnuts mixed with a small box of organic raisins

Lunch: SevenPoint2 Shake and ¾ cup mixed vegetables

Snack: 2-3 SevenPoint2 Green caps and 1 slice of watermelon ½ inch thick

Dinner: Un-spaghetti: 4-6 ounces prepared no-sugar spaghetti sauce with meat, placed on 1 cup steamed spaghetti squash, ½ cup broccoli

Snack (optional): ½ cup of sliced cucumbers with 2 tablespoons hummus

At Bedtime: Take 4 SevenPoint2 Alkaline Boosters

MAINTENANCE

You did it! You have completed the Seven-Week Transformation and may or may not be ready for a maintenance program. If you still have health goals that you would like to achieve, it is recommended that you stay on the program as long as you feel necessary. If you are ready to move to maintenance, or what SevenPoint2 refers to as a "lifetime of health," we recommend the following program:

1. One SevenPoint2 Shake per day in place of one protein serving

2. One or two servings of SevenPoint2 Greens

3. At this point, you may start to reintroduce one serving per day of grains into your diet (it is recommended to still keep these to a minimum). Ideal grains are rice, quinoa, and millet. Others (not ideal) are whole grain wheat, rye, oats, and barley.

Please Note: More details and FAQs about the Seven-Week Transformation can be found at www.SevenPoint2Transformation.com

Foods to Avoid

Definitely avoid these foods during the Seven-Week Transformation, and it is recommended to avoid them for a lifetime.

- Any food that you are — or suspect you are — allergic to
- All refined sugars
- All artificial sweeteners
- Corn syrup
- Dairy products, such as milk, cheese, yogurt, and ice

cream

- Gluten products, such as bread, pasta, and other foods made with wheat, rye, and barley[1]
- Corn and corn products
- Soy and all products made with soy
- Alcohol
- Carbonated beverages
- Peanuts and peanut butter
- Pork, cold cuts, bacon, and sausage
- Hot dogs and canned meats
- Shellfish
- Meat substitutes
- Meats that contain nitrates or nitrites
- Night shades (if you are prone to swelling or joint pain), such as tomatoes, white potatoes, eggplant, and bell peppers

[1]Wheat grass and barley grass are gluten free.

Foods to Eat

Fruit (½ cup servings)	Vegetable (1 cup servings)	Protein (3-5 ounce portions) (organic sources	Grains (½ cup servings)
Pineapple*	Spinach*	Turkey	*(Note: If you are*
Avocado	Leafy greens*	Chicken	*eating protein, do*
Lime/lemon*	Celery*	Elk-venison	*not add a grain at*
Tangerine*	Carrots*	Buffalo	*the same meal—*
Strawberries*	Asparagus*	Wild salmon	*only protein*
Grapefruit*	Cabbage*	Halibut	*and vegetables*
Apricot*	Broccoli*	Trout	*or grain and*
Blackberries*	Zucchini	Beans (Lentils*,	*vegetables)*
Raspberries*	Sweet potatoes	black-eyed*,	
Orange	(1-2 times a week)	black*, pinto*,	Quinoa
Peach*	Pumpkin*	kidney*, navy*,	Millet
Grapes*	Lettuce*	garbanzo*)	Rice
Blueberries	Kale*	Duck eggs	Buckwheat
Apple*	Brussels sprouts*	Chicken eggs	
Pear*	Bok choy	(rarely)	
Watermelon	Cauliflower*		
Nectarine*	Beets* (1-2 times	**Nuts & Seeds** (1/4 cup serving) (organic sources)	**Sweeteners** (1 tablespoon)
Plum	a week)		
Prunes*	Radishes*		
Kiwi*	Green peas	Almonds	
Papaya	Snow peas	Sunflower seeds	Molasses
Pomegranate*	Sauerkraut	Pumpkin seeds	Pure maple syrup
	Parsnips	Walnuts	Stevia
	Mushrooms		Lakanto®
	Green beans*		Xylitol
	Onion		
	Garlic		
	Artichoke*		
	Turnips*		
	Cucumber*		
	Squash*		

Other Fruits (no more than 2 times per week)	Oils (2 teaspoons)	Milk Products (non-dairy) (1 cup, unsweetened) (organic where possible)	Other Beverages
Raisins (1/4 cup) Banana (1 small) Figs (5) Dates (5 medjool) Cantaloupe * Cherries * Pineapples * Mangos *	Coconut Ghee (clarified butter) Hemp Olive	Milk substitutes only: Rice Almond Hemp Cashew Coconut	Herbal teas Alkalized water Water, water!!!
*Negative-calorie foods			

Simple Process

FIRST
Eat alkaline-forming foods in proper proportions: 80 percent alkaline to 20 percent acid-forming foods.

SECOND
When you eat an imbalanced meal, make sure that you replace your potential mineral loss with the SevenPoint2 Alkaline Booster.

THIRD
Drink at least one half to two thirds of your body weight in ounces of water per day. Ideally, you want your water to be alkaline.

FOURTH
Get moving! Log on to www.SevenPoint2Transformation.com, and follow the simple and easy workout programs that have been designed specifically to *not* overload your adrenals.

Note: This process has been described in very simple terms. If you have a health condition of any kind, please consult your health practitioner before starting any diet or exercise program.

12 Key Points

1. Eat fresh organic foods *daily*.

2. Eat nutrient rich foods. The perfect combo is SevenPoint2 Greens and Shake.

3. Eat live, raw foods (uncooked fruits and vegetables) as much as possible.

4. Keep animal protein (chicken, beef, and eggs) to a minimum. The ideal portion size would be 3-5 ounces per meal.

5. Keep stimulants and stimulant drinks (coffee, cola, green/black tea, refined sugar, and chocolate) to a minimum (small amounts of premium dark chocolate are okay occasionally: 1 serving per week).

6. Drink at least one half to two thirds of your body weight in ounces of water per day (alkaline is ideal)

7. Eat only healthy fats, like almonds, flax, hemp, avocado, or coconut.

8. Get a good night's sleep.

9. Learn techniques to help reduce stress in your life.

10. Exercise a few times a week (both cardio and strength).

11. Do something that brings you joy each day.

12. *Make a difference in someone's life.* Help them to get healthy by sharing the SevenPoint2 Seven Week Alkaline Transformation program so they, too, can enjoy the health and vitality benefits of an alkaline lifestyle.

SevenPoint2 Product Line

SevenPoint2 Recovery with HydroFX™

Recovery with HydroFX™ is comprised of a unique blend of redox-active, hydrogen-generating, alkaline minerals. This breakthrough proprietary formula has been clinically tested to release molecular hydrogen; produce a negative oxidation reduction potential; create an antacid, alkalizing effect; and increase cellular hydration. The most notable benefit is its ability to release such a significant amount of molecular hydrogen (H2).

Recovery with HydroFX™ is alkalizing. It effectively neutralizes excess acids, including lactic acid, in bodies of all types.

Helps to:

- Reduce inflammation
- Reduce joint discomfort
- Reduce lactic acid
- Increase energy
- Anti-aging
- Cardio-protective
- Neuro-protective
- Intestinal protection
- Skin rejuvenation
- Increase stamina
- And much more*

"As a personal trainer, working out is my livelihood. After taking Recovery regularly, the pain of lactic acid building up is no longer a deterrent to my workouts. My bounce-back time is back to where it was in my early twenties. This product rocks!"*—Mike Z.

SevenPoint2 Shake

The great tasting vegan shake is the foundation of your alkaline lifestyle. The SevenPoint2™ Shake's proprietary formula is an excellent high-quality/low-carbohydrate protein source. This easily digestible formula is high in fiber and provides an extensive array of naturally occurring amino acids, which are the building blocks of protein. This low-glycemic/high-performance vegetarian superfood assists your body in burning fat and becoming alkaline, all at the same time.

- Organic
- Vegan
- Kosher
- Sugar free
- Non-GMO
- Gluten free
- Soy free
- Dairy free
- Nut free

"This is by far the best-tasting shake I have ever had. It is so clean with regards to the ingredients. I took it in for my family doctor to see, and he was impressed."* —Laura H.

SevenPoint2 Greens

SevenPoint2™ Organic Greens are a delicious and revitalizing essential supplement designed to gently detoxify the body and help you achieve an alkaline lifestyle.

Our greens are loaded with healthy green superfoods, cereal grasses, and alkalizing vegetables in a great-tasting powder. Unlike other green products commonly associated with an unfavorable taste, our greens taste so good that even the most finicky palates will enjoy them. They really do taste that good.

"These are the best-tasting greens. My entire family loves them, and that makes me feel better, especially since it's hard to get our children to eat lots of greens. SevenPoint2 Greens provide the best nutrition for us all."* — Brooke B.

SevenPoint2 Green Caps

The SevenPoint2 Green Caps are a revitalizing essential supplement designed to feed your body the nutrients it needs and to help you achieve an alkaline lifestyle. The Green caps are loaded with plenty of healthy green superfoods, cereal grasses, and alkalizing vegetables.

- Contain only organic ingredients
- One hundred percent whole-food, non-GMO, vegan nutrition
- Convenient, easy-to-swallow capsule
- Naturally energizing
- Certified kosher
- Gluten free, dairy free, soy free, nut free, nightshade free, sugar free, and free of all artificial ingredients

"I've been working two jobs and am usually exhausted by three o'clock in the afternoon. Since I started taking the SevenPoint2 Green Caps, I've been full of energy, I have more mental clarity, and my cravings for sweets and coffee have vanished! It's unbelievable! Thanks SevenPoint2."* — Robert F., Chicago, IL

SevenPoint2 Alkaline Booster

We have affectionately nicknamed our Alkaline Booster, "The Hall Pass." After having an acidic meal and/or beverage(s), or before bed, this product works instantly to bring you from acidic pH levels to alkaline. The SevenPoint2™ Alkaline Booster allows you to live the lifestyle you are accustomed to, while staying on track with your goal of being pH balanced.

"For years, I've had major digestive issuesthat have really affected my life. I noticed a huge improvement in just a couple of days using these Alkaline Boosters. I love them and take them every day."* —Jason M.

*These statements have not been evaluated by the Food and Drug Administration. This product is not intended to diagnose, treat, cure, or prevent any disease.

Follow this program the way it is designed, and watch your life transform.

Personal Success Agreement:

One of the most important parts of any successful program is the commitment to doing your absolute best throughout the process. Starting a new health program can be exciting, but what people sometimes forget is that getting healthy is a process that takes time, and the results are not always immediate. Making the commitment to follow through with the entire program takes real dedication to yourself, as does remembering why you started the program in the first place.

My reason for starting the program:

_____

(Examples: weight loss, self-image, health concerns, freedom to do what I want)

I, _____, commit—to myself and to those I love—to become a healthier and more vibrant person by bringing my body into a more balanced and healthy pH. I know that I may feel restricted, but I also know that the process of learning and enjoying new and healthy food habits takes time, and as my body heals, I will crave the new, healthier foods over the unhealthy ones. I may want to give in to unhealthy food choices, but instead I will ask for help when I need support.

I am committing to the SevenPoint2 Seven-Week Alkaline Transformation for better health and therefore a better life. I DESERVE IT!

_____ Signature

_____ Date

For more information about the SevenPoint2 Seven-Week Alkaline Transformation and the SevenPoint2 Product Line, go to www.SevenPoint2.com.

Be Well—Go Alkaline

Now that we have created a winning strategy that anyone can follow with diet and nutrition, we need to say a few words about what many experts believe to be our greatest acidifier—stress. In fact, when speaking to patients about the adrenal glands, most physiciansdescribe them as the "stress glands." When we think of stress, we usually think of emotional stress; however, stress can also come from physical, as well as chemical and environmental, factors. When we are really stressed, we are often described as "hot." Heat equals inflammation, and inflammation equals acidity. Managing stress is also vitally important in attaining and maintaining an alkaline body.

So, what have we learned in this chapter? First, we are living in a world that is undergoing an acid crisis. Second, moving towards an alkaline lifestyle greatly improves our chances for good health. Lastly, better ways now exist to make it simple, easy, cost-effective, and palatable to maintain the proper diet, so that anyone can become alkaline.

I will leave you with this chilling thought: It has been said that the average person in America spends more money in their last two weeks of life on trying to stay alive than they do in their *whole* life on prevention. There is an old Chinese proverb that states, "Don't wait until you're thirsty to dig a well," which, in this case, means that it's a whole lot easier to stay well than it is to get well.

Darien

When she was only twelve years old, my daughter, Darien, had migraines. She saw many doctors, starting with the pediatrician. She was on home and hospital teaching; she couldn't attend school.

Her doctors were convinced that she was depressed and basically crazy. They had given her a billion tests. They did blood work, allergy tests, brain scans—all kinds of stuff. We had to see a psychiatrist for the depression, which only made her feel crazy. They put her on so many medicines— first antidepressants and then pills to counteract the effects of the antidepressants. They just over-medicated her.

When Darien told me that she had given up on life, I made them take her off of all the antidepressants. That was when my cousin sent me an email from her cousin, who was a patient of Dr. Zodkoy. I made the appointment, and we were there three days later.

Within one week of being on Dr. Zodkoy's adrenal fatigue program, Darien was my kid again. She was practically back to normal. It was amazing. It gives me goose bumps to talk about it. She got out of bed. She wanted to go back to school. It was phenomenal. I didn't have to worry about what could possibly be wrong with my kid any more. I could sleep at night.

Dr. Zodkoy saved my daughter's life in more ways than one. His adrenal fatigue program gave her her life back and allowed her to be a normal twelve year old. It also enabled her to release the extra weight she had been carrying for years. (She had always been forty to fifty pounds overweight and could never lose weight.)

When she walked into high school at fourteen years old, Darien was down from a size 7 to a size 3, and her friends didn't recognize her. She became a social butterfly, made new friends, and got a boyfriend.

Now she's twenty and in college. Dr. Zodkoy's program has allowed her to continue down the right path. It gave her confidence.

Conclusion

This book was a labor of love for me, because I find writing to be an extremely difficult task, but I felt that the information was too important not to share it. Adrenal fatigue is an epidemic that is crippling America and is going unnoticed by most physicians, so it is going to be up to the general public to seek out proper care.My goal for this book was to help those who have not gotten the right care for their health complaints by guiding them to the road less traveled, which, as in other areas of life, often offers the solution.

I believe that adrenal fatigue is a major cause of many of today's health issues — including anxiety, depression, PTSD, fibromyalgia, and chronic pain — and should be considered as a diagnosis for anyone who has not received the care and relief that they deserve. The adrenal fatigue diagnosis explains why patients have both physical and emotional complaints which do not respond to traditional care, and it offers hope to those who need it the most. The fact that so many of my patients with "untreatable" conditions have recovered by following the adrenal fatigue treatment protocol demonstrates that there is hope. While the advancements in medical testing of cortisol levels, DHEA, and neurotransmitters have made it easier to properly diagnose adrenal fatigue, the treatment has remained the same.

Treating adrenal fatigue requires the patient to attack the problem on both an emotional and a physical level. Adrenal fatigue treatment will only be effective when a patient can deal with the emotional and physical stressors that brought the condition out and then dedicate themself to rebuilding themself physically and emotionally. Thisprovides an opportunity for a person to reset their lifestyle and learn to put themself first.

Many adrenal fatigue sufferers learn to see their condition as a blessing,changing their lives from stress and excess to rest and accepting their best.

I want to thank you for reading my book and to leave you with the toast that the wisest man in the world, my father, used for forty years.

"I wish you health, wealth, and the time to enjoy it." — Mel Zodkoy (1930-1994)

Wishing you good health,
Dr. Steven Zodkoy

About the Author

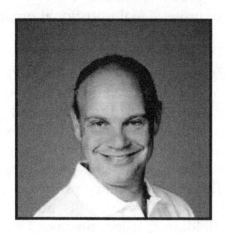

Dr. Steven Zodkoy, DC, CNS, DACBN, DABCN

Dr. Steven Zodkoy is a board-certified chiropractor, nutritionist, and kinesiologist who, for over twenty years, has specialized in treating patients who have been deemed "untreatable" through a standard course of treatment. Dr. Zodkoy attended Rutgers University and received his bachelor's degree and Doctor of Chiropractic degree from Los Angeles College of Chiropractic at the age of twenty-four. He is currently a licensed chiropractor in the states of New Jersey and New York and the Commonwealth of Pennsylvania. Dr. Zodkoy is an applied kinesiologist, Certified Nutrition Specialist® (CNS®), a Diplomate of the Chiropractic Board of Clinical Nutrition (DCBCN) and a Diplomate of the American Clinical Board of Nutrition (DACBN).

Dr. Zodkoy is a leader in his field. He was the first chiropractor to pass the American College of Nutrition (ACN) exam given by the Certification Board for Nutrition Specialists (CBNS), an organization which had previously been limited to medical doctors and PhDs. Dr. Zodkoy has been a nutritional consultant to the New Jersey Chiropractic Association and was instrumental in helping to achieve a new scope of practice for New Jersey Chiropractors. He also developed and organized one of the largest professional nutritional organizations in the country.

Currently, Dr. Zodkoy has a practice in Freehold, New Jersey and is active in medical research for the United States military. He believes that education to the public and professionals is the best way to promote health. He regularly lectures to groups in his community, speaks at corporate events, and holds continuing education courses for medical professionals.He presently is working with military personnel and veterans to overcome the effects of PTSD and TBIs, and his recent research into this area is yielding excellent results.

"There are no untreatable patients, just untried treatments." — Dr. Steven Zodkoy

Reference Information

Specific Nutritional Supplements for Specific Issues

Adrenal fatigue sufferers have numerous symptoms and complaints, which is why they often get misdiagnosed, but the symptoms and complaints all have the same underlying cause. When I treat a patient in my office or around the world, the first nutritional supplements I recommend are designed to support and rebuild the adrenal glands. These core nutritional supplements are the same for almost everyone. Remember that with adrenal fatigue, the symptoms may be different, but the cause is the same. The second set of nutrients I recommend are those that will help alleviate the most serious complaints and aid in their recovery. It is neither necessary nor advisable to treat every symptom. As the adrenal glands heal, most complaints will abate.

There are a variety of nutritional companies that provide adrenal support products. I have yet to find the perfect product or product line. I have found the most success when I combine a number of different products from several different vendors. The quality of nutritional products varies greatly among companies and directly affects how well the body responds to them. The products mentioned on the following pages have been tested to ensure the highest quality ingredients, proper potency, purity, and absorption, while eliminating artificial ingredients, allergens, and toxins.

Most of the nutrients listed are exactly what I recommend for my own patients. These products are the best of the best, designed to balance the body so that it may heal properly. Do not confuse these nutritional supplements with franchise brands. Yes, they are both nutritional supplements but only in the sense that "chicken nuggets" are in the same realm as organic chicken breast. Chicken nuggets do contain chicken, but how much, what else, and how were they made? These are not questions you should have about your food or your nutritional supplements.

Many of these products can only be ordered through a physician or physician's website and can be difficult to find in just one place. I have simplified the ordering process by allowing you to order nutritional supplements through Doctors Supplement Store, an independent company that has all the necessary products in one place. You can order on the internetor by phone, and you will need to give them my name, Dr. Zodkoy, and code SZ400.

www.DSSorders.com/drzodkoy
877-846-7122

This website is restricted, so remember to enter in Dr. Zodkoy and Code: SZ400

I am presently working on my own line of nutritional supplements to address adrenal fatigue. These nutritional supplements are based on the successful formulas I have used to treat military personnel. Please check out my website to learn more. A portion of the sales of these nutrients will be donated to treating veterans and active duty personnel with adrenal fatigue.

www.TheAdrenalFatigueLink.com

Adrenal fatigue core nutrients have been chosen to work together to rebuild the adrenal glands and energize the mind and body. When taken regularly, patients often feel a dramatic change in just a few weeks.

Adrenal Fatigue Core Nutrients

1. **Ortho Molecular — Adren-All, 120 Capsules**
   This is an adrenal-gland-based supplement that is excellent for fatigue and pain.*

2. **Innate Response Formulas — Adrenal Response® Complete Care**
   This adaptogen-herbal-based nutritional product is excellent for supporting the adrenal glands' rebuilding and production. It also tends to have a relaxing and calming effect.*

3. **Ortho Molecular — Alpha Base Foundation Pak, 60 Packets**
   This is a multi-nutrient product that supplies vitamins, minerals, essential oils, phytonutrients, and probiotics. It is easy to digest and is a key component to the program.*

Nutritional Supplements for Specific Symptoms

You may add the following nutrients to the adrenal fatigue core nutrients based on your worst one or two symptoms. *Do not try to treat every symptom.* Remember that treating adrenal fatigue is about rebuilding the adrenal glands, which in turn will reduce your symptoms and complaints. The suggestions below are designed to help ease your worst symptoms while the adrenals rebuild.

Anxiety:

Mild: Designs for Health — NeuroCalm™*
Severe: Neuroscience, Inc. — Kavinace*

Asthma/Bronchitis:

Thorne Research — T.Asthmatica Plus®*

Burnout:

NeuroScience, Inc. — Kavinace*
Allergy Research Group — DHEA 50 mg Micronized Lipid Matrix*

Blood Sugar/Glucose Problems:

Allergy Research Group — Sugar Balance Formula*

Dizziness:

Integrative Therapeutics — Ginkgo Biloba Plus*

Erectile Dysfunction or Poor Male Libido:

Designs for Health — LibidoStim-M™*

Fatigue:

Designs for Health — CoQnol™(Ubiquinol-Reduced CoQ10) 100mg*

Fibromyalgia:

Designs for Health — SAMe 400mg, Blister Pack, 30 tablets*

GI Issues:

Ortho Molecular — Ortho Biotic*

Headache:

Thorne Research — Neurochondria®*

Hot Flashes/Menopause:

Allergy Research Group—DHEA 50 mg Micronized Lipid Matrix*
Vital Nutrients—Menopause Support*

Immune System Weakness:

Designs for Health—Immunitone Plus™*

Insomnia:

NeuroScience, Inc.—Kavinace Ultra PM*

Migraines:

Thorne Research—T.A.P.S.®*
Thorne Research—Neurochondria®*

Neuropathy:

Thorne Research—Neurochondria®*

Pain—Joint/Muscles/Inflammation:

Thorne Research—Ar-Encap®*

PTSD:

DHEA 100mg*

Urination—Frequent or Incontinence:

Thorne Research—Uristatin®*

*These statements have not been evaluated by the Food and Drug Administration. This product is not intended to diagnose, treat, cure, or prevent any disease.

Questions and Answers

Q: Why didn't you include any research or references in the book?

A: The computer age has made the inclusion of research unnecessary and inefficient. There is an unlimited amount of information available online which can offer multiple viewpoints to an issue. If you are interested in reading the research that my book is based on, I would encourage you to go to www.PubMed.com. PubMed is part of the United States National Library of Medicine (NLM), National Institutes of Health (NIH). PubMed compiles medical research articles from around the world into a very useable search engine. There are also links to research articles on my website at www. TheAdrenalFatigueLink.com.

Q: Where can I find a doctor who can diagnose and treat adrenal fatigue?

A: The International College of Applied Kinesiology website at www.ICAK.com is an excellent place to begin your search for a physician who can diagnose and treat adrenal fatigue.

Q: Where can I find a Doctor who practices Neuro Emotional Technique?

A: The NET website at www.NETMindBody.com has more information and a list of physicians.

Q: Where can I order an Alpha-Stim® unit?
A: www.Alpha-Stim.com

Q: Where can I learn more about an alkaline diet and alkaline products?
A: http://stevez.sevenpoint2.com/

Made in the USA
Las Vegas, NV
28 August 2023

76756649R10125